EXTRAPYRAMIDAL DISORDERS IN CHILDHOOD

EXTRAPYRAMIDAL DISORDERS IN CHILDHOOD

Proceedings of the Postgraduate Course on Extrapyramidal
Diseases in Childhood held in Pavia, Italy, 14–15 May 1987

Editors:

Lucia Angelini
Department of Child Neurology
Istituto Neurologico 'C. Besta',
Milano, Italy

Umberto Balottin
Department of Child Neurology
Istituto Neurologico 'C. Mondino',
University of Pavia, Pavia, Italy

Giovanni Lanzi
Department of Child Neurology
Istituto Neurologico 'C. Mondino',
University of Pavia, Pavia, Italy

Nardo Nardocci
Department of Child Neurology
Istituto Neurologico 'C. Besta',
Milano, Italy

 1987

EXCERPTA MEDICA, Amsterdam–New York–Oxford

International Congress Series No. 746
ISBN 0 444 80919 8

Published by:
Elsevier Science Publishers B.V. (Biomedical Division)
P.O. Box 211
1000 AE Amsterdam
The Netherlands

Sole distributors for the USA and Canada:
Elsevier Science Publishing Company Inc.
52 Vanderbilt Avenue
New ork, NY 10017
USA

Printed in The Netherlands

Preface

It is my privilege to introduce this volume which reports the Proceedings of the Meeting on Extrapyramidal Disorders in Childhood held in Pavia, May 1987.

The subject represents a main topic in child neurology because of the problems of nosographic systemization and consequently of diagnosis, prognosis and therapy.

The volume includes reports on the different aspects of the extrapyramidal disorders with a close interrelation between the basic and clinical neurosciences. I trust that this volume will be a helpful reference for those interested in child neurology.

Professor Renato Boeri
Scientific Director

Introduction

Movement disorders have become significantly interesting as a subject in the Neurosciences. The majority of the data, however, relate to the more specific problems of extrapyramidal disorders in adults. As a disease in childhood it still remains poorly systemized.

This book is a collection of certain studies with reference to the most recent advances regarding the morphofunctional organization of the basal ganglia in relation to development. Moreover, the book attempts to systemize the extrapyramidal diseases typical of childhood or at the onset in childhood, focusing on diagnostic and therapeutic criteria.

The Meeting on the Extrapyramidal Disorders was supported by the Fondazione Pierfranco Mariani and the Proceedings by the Istituto Neurologico 'C. Besta' of Milan.

We have a particular debt to the Istituto Neurologico 'C. Mondino' and The University of Pavia for their good cooperation and we thank Dr. Marina Bentivoglio and Dr. Roberto Spreafico for their helpful suggestions in preparing the Meeting.

The Editors

Contents

© 1987 Elsevier Science Publishers B.V. (Biomedical Division)
Extrapyramidal disorders in childhood
L. Angelini et al. editors

1

ONTOGENY OF DOPAMINERGIC AND CHOLINERGIC SYSTEMS IN THE BASAL
GANGLIA

ANN M. GRAYBIEL and HELEN NEWMAN-GAGE

Department of Brain and Cognitive Sciences, Massachusetts
Institute of Technology, Cambridge, Massachusetts 02139

At birth, the human brain is far from fully developed and
much evidence now suggests that modeling of neural connections on
the basis of experience is a crucial aspect of postnatal
maturation. The neurobiology of this early postnatal
"plasticity" has been intensively studied for the visual system,
in which a variety of experimental manipulations of the inputs
are straightforward. In this system, it is known that both
selective retraction of collaterals or entire processes and
neuronal cell death, as well as formation of new sprouts and
synaptic connections underlie these critical developmental
changes (1). Far less is known about the neural basis of
maturation and plasticity in the central motor system, even
though at the behavioral level the gradual development of normal
movement patterns is perhaps the most obvious and well-
documented aspect of postnatal maturation, and, at the cellular
level, the development of the peripheral motor neuronal synapse,
the neuromuscular junction, is a premier model of synaptogenesis
(2).

For the motor system, classic studies have emphasized the
prolonged maturation time of the cerebral cortex and of cortical
efferent pathways such as the pyramidal tract as keys to
understanding normal motor development. However, the important
influence of extrapyramidal systems on the control of motor
behaviors (as demonstrated by the striking deficits of conditions
such as Huntington's chorea and Parkinson's disease) underscores
the significance of maturational features within the
extrapyramidal as well as the directly descending pyramidal
systems. We here briefly review evidence suggesting that
remarkably extensive changes occur in subcortical parts of the
motor system in concert with the postnatal development of normal

movement patterns. In particular, we will focus on changes in the cholinergic neurons of the basal ganglia and in the related dopamine-containing nuclei of the nigral complex.

Major components of basal ganglia circuitry include the caudate nucleus and putamen (collectively known as the striatum), the globus pallidus (with its internal and external segments) and the substantia nigra and subthalamic nucleus, two nuclei tightly interlinked with the striatum and pallidum (3,4,5). Altogether, these regions are interconnected through a complex series of loops whose final summated output is carried by way of pallidothalamic and nigrothalamic pathways in turn leading to premotor and supplementary motor cortex. These cortical areas, in turn, project to the motor cortex (area 4) and themselves have descending connections as well. The main input side of this basal ganglia system--though not the only input station--is the striatum, which receives forebrain afferents from the cortex, the thalamus and the amygdala as well as ascending afferents from the midbrain, principally from the dopamine-containing nigral complex. For each class of afferent connection there is a broad division between inputs to the "dorsal striatum" (caudate nucleus and putamen of classic descriptions) and inputs to the "ventral striatum" (nucleus accumbens and related regions). The ventral striatal afferents are generally categorized as being related to the limbic system (e.g., inputs from the hippocampus and from the midline and paramedian dopamine-containing neurons of the midbrain's ventral tegmental area).

Unlike the thalamus, the striatum does not have direct reciprocal connections with the cortex. Rather, it appears to be the inlet to a complex processing unit, the subcortical forebrain extrapyramidal system. The massive efferent projections from the striatum lead not only to the globus pallidus but also to the substantia nigra pars reticulata, the non-dopaminergic part of the nigral complex and, in lesser volume, to the dopamine-containing substantia nigra pars compacta. The nigrostriatal tract, carrying dopamine to the striatum, completes a loop back to the striatum and again, a parallel pathway, known as the mesolimbic tract, exists for the limbic striatum. Now differentiated as a separate dopamine-containing system is the pathway from the caudal nigral complex ("cell group A8") to the striatum.

These mesostriatal pathways are singularly important in extrapyramidal motor control. It is well-known that degeneration of dopaminergic nigrostriatal neurons results in the hallmark parkinsonian symptoms of bradykinesia, tremor, and rigidity. The added clinical finding that anticholinergic drugs provide some symptomatic relief, coupled with findings in physiologic studies in animals led to the hypothesis of a dopaminergic/cholinergic balance in the striatum, and suggested that perturbations in this balance occur in disease states (6,7,8,9).

In addition to its looping interconnections, a second order of complexity in the striatum has relatively recently been discovered. At first glance, a histologic section shows the caudate and putamen and even the substantia nigra to be rather homogeneous nuclei. However, many studies employing immunohistochemical markers for transmitter-related substances, as well as anterograde and retrograde axon transport studies, have revealed that a complex compartmentalized architecture exists within the striatum (10,11). Principal elements of this compartmental arechitecture are the striosomes (striatal bodies). These appear in serial coronal section reconstructions to be tubular, branched structures (0.3-0.5 mm in diameter) that traverse the striatum to form a rostrocaudally and mediolaterally directed labyrinth. Nearly every neurotransmitter-related substance so far localized to the striatum follows a striosomal ordering. This is true for the human striatum as well as for striatal tissue from every other mammalian species so far studied.

The striosomes were first demonstrated with a histochemical stain for acetylcholinesterase (AChE), the degredative enzyme of the cholinergic synapse (12). The same distribution has now been shown for the catabolic cholinergic enzyme, choline acetyltransferase (9). In tissue sections, the striosomes appear as circumscribed macroscopic patches of low AChE activity embedded in a matrix of concentrated AChE activity. Correlative studies of sections immunohistochemically or autoradiographically treated so as to demonstrate other neurotransmitter-related substances have since shown inhomogeneities of distribution in patterns identical or nearly identical to that of the AChE-poor striosomes. This is not only true for the cholinergic and dopaminergic marker enzymes marking the locations of the cholinergic interneurons of the striatum and its dopamine-containing afferents (13), but is also true for many neuropeptides such as substance P, NT, NPY, SOM, enkephalin and dynorphin, and for a number of receptor-related binding sites including muscarinic cholinergic and D_1 and D_2 dopaminergic ligand binding sites (10,11,14,15). There thus appears to be an architectural framework for the crucial balance of dopaminergic and cholinergic regulation in the striatum, but also an accompanying architecture in register with this for the other transmitter-related substances of the striatum. There is no doubt that this broader view of the organization of the cholinergic-dopaminergic elements of the striatum, which places them in the context of other transmitter-coded systems, will help in understanding how an imbalance between acetylcholine- and dopamine-mediated processing can result in a variety of abnormal conditions, one example of which is Parkinson's disease.

Studies of the ontogeny of the striatum show that this architecture undergoes remarkable transformations in order to finally achieve its characteristic adult form. One might expect a gradual increase in background matrix staining of tissue surrounding ever paler-appearing striosomes. However, this is not the case. In the human fetus (and other fetal mammals), the future striosomes are the most intensely AChE-stained structures of the developing striatum. These striking, densely-stained inhomogeneities are coextensive with the regions refered to in the developing brain as dopamine islands because they were first histochemically identified as regions of intense catecholamine (mainly dopamine)-induced fluorescence (16,17). We now know that the dopamine islands are collections of early-arriving dopamine-containing fibers originating in the substantia nigra pars compacta. That the dopamine islands are also islands of intense

AChE staining probably reflects the presence of AChE as well as dopamine in these fibers.

From study of very young fetal brains (in the cat) it is becomming clear that the dopamine islands are key foci in the early development of the striatum (4). With the aid of antibodies that detect synaptic vesicle protein, it has been shown by light and electron microscopy that the dopamine islands are the sites of early, concentrated synaptogenesis in the striatum (18,19). Also, in intrauterine axon transport studies (in the rat), it has been found that neurons in the regions innervated by dopamine island fibers are probably the first striatal cells to project to the substantia nigra (20,21).

The fetal pattern of intensely staining AChE-positive patches in a pale matrix is the exact reverse of that found in adulthood. There is excellent evidence that the reversal in patterning actually occurs--i.e., that the AChE-rich patches of the fetal striatum will become the AChE-poor zones at adulthood. Techniques that radioactively label the DNA of dividing cells (^{3}H-thymidine autoradiography) permanently mark such cells. With these methods it has been shown that nerve cells of the fetal dopamine island regions are indeed the cells that occupy the adult striosomes (22). These studies have also documented that the island neurons are generated early, before most neurons of the surrounding matrix.

This architectural continuity points to the establishment of the modular organization of the striatum early on during development. Consonant with this idea is evidence that during development many other transmitter-related substances, including receptor ligands and neurotransmitters also come to have distributions respecting the dopamine island/striosome borders. The particular time of onset of the modular rearrangements varies with the substance and its exact locale in the striatum. The consistent and early developmental compartmentalization underscores the basic significance of the dopamine island/striosome system, with the dopamine islands representing the focal point of change. The mediatiors of the differential and changing distributions most likely include not only extrinsic afferents (including the dopamine-island fibers themselves) but also intrinsically-timed expression of neurotransmitter-related features endogenous to developing striatal neurons.

From the standpoint of clinical studies, it is of great interest that the transition from an immature to mature striatal architecture occurs postnatally for most of these neurotransmitter-related compounds. In the human, the transition from AChE-rich to AChE-poor striosomes occurs during the first months of life (23). For comparison, this change occurs during the first weeks of life in the cat, and during about the first month of life in rodents (22,24). The distribution of AChE staining in the newborn child resembles that of the fetus in that there are AChE-rich islands in a less intensely stained matrix. Such AChE-positive islands are still visible at three months, but in the brain of a single 3.5 month old child (23) the transition was clearly underway in that AChE-poor zones had begun to appear.

It is important to keep in mind that the gradual disappearance of the AChE-rich islands--and appearance of AChE-poor striosomes--not only implies that there has been a change in the islandic/striosomal regions, but also that there has been a change in the AChE staining of the matrix. As mentioned above, AChE staining of the dopamine islands may actually reflect AChE contained within or at least specifically associated with the dopamine-containing fibers. Recent experiments with ^{3}H hemicholinium however, suggests that these AChE-positive patches may also be indicative of cholinergic processes (25). There is no doubt that most of the AChE staining that later develops in the extrastriosomal matrix accurately reflects cholinergic processes (9). Thus, it is virtually certain that during the perinatal and early postnatal period there is a sharp increase in the cholinergic innervation of the matrix relative to that of the striosomes.

In terms of the functional significance of these shifts, it is remarkable that in concert, there are radical shifts in the distribution of muscarinic receptor binding sites of the M_1 and

M_2 types both in the human and in the (more systematically studied) cat (26,27). Apparently, a parallel change takes place in the dopamine-containing fibers of the striosomes and matrix, at least insofar as they can be tracked through development with tyrosine hydroxylase immunohistochemistry (22). The dopamine islands, originally vivid tyrosine hydroxylase-positive islands in a tyrosine hydroxylase-poor matrix, give way to become zones relatively impoverished in tyrosine hydroxylase by comparison with the extrastriosomal matrix (13).

During the transitional phase for the distributions of these cholinergic and dopaminergic markers, the clearly defined, well-structured modular ordering characteristic of the fetal striatum appears to become chaotic. AChE staining intensifies in the matrix areas but the entire striatum takes on a marbled appearance and whereas some pale AChE-poor striosomes can be found, distinct AChE-rich islands can still be identified as well. The different character of the patches follows a developmental topography, as do the equally difficult-to-follow changes in muscarinic cholinergic ligand binding. The distribution of dopamine-containing fibers comes to include more and more the matrix. From work on nigrostriatal connectivity, it now seems likely that these changes reflect different rates of development of subsystems within the mesostriatal projection (28,29). Interestingly, in the cat at least, the tyrosine hydroxylase-rich dopamine islands can be seen with immunohistochemistry later than the heightened AChE staining of the islands. It is as though the AChE changes were lagging, by a small interval, the changes in dopamine-containing innervation. In time, however, the cholinergic neurons of the striatum undergo a spurt of development especially, it seems, in the extrastriosomal matrix.

Though the postnatal schedules of cholinergic and dopaminergic development may not be in complete synchrony, it appears likely that the expansion of dopamine-containing fibers into the extrastriosomal matrix regions is linked to the development of the intrinsic cholinergic system of the striatum. Indirect evidence supporting this postulated linkage comes from experiments in which intrastriatal grafts of fetal striatal primordia into ibotinic-acid lesioned host striatum (in rats) have been shown to express both tyrosine hydroxylase immunoreactivity (indicative of innervation by host dopamine-containing fibers) and choline acetyltransferase-like immunoreactivity indicative of the presence of cholinergic neurons and their processes in cells and neuropil in the same patchy regions of the grafts (30).

In light of human disease states where imbalance of dopaminergic and cholinergic mechanisms seems to be responsible for part or even much of the motor symptomology, it seems highly likely that the postnatal schedules of development of the cholinergic and dopaminergic mechansims within the striatum play a role in the developing sophistication of motor behaviors in the human infant.

ACKNOWLEDGEMENTS

We thank the Seaver Institute, the McKnight Foundation and NSF BNS 8319547 for support.

REFERENCES

1. Lund RD (1978) In: Development and Plasticity of the Brain. Oxford University Press, New York, pp 183-284

2. Purves D, Lichtman JW (1985) In: Principles of Neural Development. Sinauer Assoc., Inc., Sunderland, Massachusetts, pp 205-228

3. Graybiel AM, Ragsdale Jr CW (1979) Prog in Brain Res 51:239-283

4. Graybiel AM (1984) In: Evered D, O'Connor M (eds) Functions of the Basal Ganglia. Ciba Foundation Symposium 107, Pitman, London, pp 114-149

5. Alexander GE, DeLong MR, Strick PL (1986) Ann Rev Neurosci 9:357-381

6. Barbeau A (1962) J Med Ass Can 87:802-807

7. Duvoisin RC (1967) Archs Neurol 17:124-136

8. McGeer PL, Boulding JE, Gibson WC, Foulkes RG (1961) J Med

Ass Am 177:665-670

9. Graybiel AM, Baughman RW, Eckenstein F (1986) Nature 323:625-627

10. Graybiel AM (1986) In: Martin JB, Barchas JD (eds) Neuropeptides in Neurologic and Psychiatric Disease. Raven Press, New York, pp 135-161

11. Graybiel AM, Ragsdale Jr CW (1983) In: Emson PC (ed) Chemical Neuroanatomy, Raven Press, New York, pp 454-463

12. Graybiel AM, Ragsdale Jr CW (1978) Proc Natl Acad Sci USA 75:5723-5726

13. Graybiel AM, Hirsch EC, Agid YA (1987) Proc Natl Acad Sci USA 84:303-307

14. Joyce JN, Sapp DW, Marshall JF (1986) Proc Natl Acad Sci USA 83:8002-8006

15. Besson M-J, Graybiel AM, Nastuk MA (1987) in progress

16. Olson L, Seiger A, Fuxe K (1972) Brain Res 44:283-288

17. Tennyson VM, Barrett RE, Cohen G, Cote L, Heikkila R, Mytilineou C (1972) Brain Res 46:251-285

18. Newman-Gage H, Graybiel AM (1986) Soc Neurosci Abstr 12:1326

19. Newman-Gage H, Graybiel AM, Matthew WD (1986) Intnl Basal Ganglia Society Symposium 2:30

20. Fishell G, van der Kooy D (1985) Soc Neurosci Abstr 11:1163

21. Fishell G, van der Kooy D (1987) J Neurosci in press

22. Graybiel AM (1984) Neuroscience 13:1157-1187

23. Graybiel AM, Ragsdale Jr CW (1980) Proc Natl Acad Sci USA 77:1214-1218

24. Kent JL, Pert CB, Herkenham M (1982) Devel Brain Res 2:487-504

25. Lowenstein PR, Slesinger PA, Singer HS, Walker LC, Casanova MF, Price DL, Coyle JT (1987) Soc Neurosci Abstr 12:1230

26. Nastuk MA, Graybiel AM (1985) Soc Neurosci Abstr 11:204

27. Nastuk MA, Graybiel AM (1985) J Comp Neurol 237:176-194

28. Graybiel AM (1986) In: Fahn S (ed) Recent Developments in Parkinson's Disease. Raven Press, New York

29. Jiminez-Castellanos J, Graybiel AM (1987) Neuroscience in press

30. Graybiel AM, Dunnett SB, Baughman RW, Liu F-C (1987) Second World Congress of Neuroscience in press

© 1987 Elsevier Science Publishers B.V. (Biomedical Division)
Extrapyramidal disorders in childhood
L. Angelini et al. editors

BASAL GANGLIA: ASPECTS OF PHYSIOLOGY AND PATHOPHYSIOLOGY

M. FORNARELLI, E. OLIVIER, P.J. DELWAIDE
Section of Neurology and Clinical Neurophysiology, University of Liege,
Hôpital de Bavière, 4020 Liege (Belgium)

The physiology of the basal ganglia is still poorly understood and subject of controversies. So, it is not surprising that the data regarding functional development in terms of age are very rare.

The physiological understanding is made complex by the different anatomo-functional role which these structures have in the phylogenetic scale. This has privilegiated the studies on primates and on Parkinson's Disease which constitutes the best available human model of basal ganglia dysfunction.

Most of concepts and notions contained in this work are taken from the more extensive reviews of De Long & Georgopoulos (1), Brooks (2), Marsden (3), Delwaide and Gonce (4) to which the reader is referred for further clarifications.

In the first section of this work, the results deriving from the fundamental neurophysiological approach will be reported. In the second section, the pathophysiology of some signs deriving from basal ganglia dysfunctions in man will be discussed highlighting the current contribution offered both by the behavioural studies and the clinical neurophysiology techniques.

CLASSICAL NEUROPHYSIOLOGY

Although the basal ganglia may play a role in other aspects of behaviour such as the language (5), the bulk of our knowledge concerns their contribution in motor control.

Motor effects of lesions

a) Globus pallidus

This nucleus constitutes, together with the pars reticulata of the substantia nigra the output component of the basal ganglia. Different authors (6,7,8) have destroyed this nucleus electrolytically. Unilateral lesions result in no obvious motor effect, while bilateral lesions produce only a transient mild hypotonia.

On the other hand, Denny Brown (9) found that larger lesions encroaching upon adjacent structures, lead to complex motor abnormalities such as akinesia, rigidity, flexion postures.

In these experiments, it is not clear whether the motor effects are due to the destruction of cells or to damage of axonal pathways; to solve that problem, more selective methods like cooling or infusion of kainic acid have been employed. Cooling blocks the synaptic transmission reversibly and kainic acid destroys cells; both methods spare axons. Hore et al. (10) found in monkeys that cooling of pallidum impairs self-paced, not visually guided movements, but has no obvious effect on movements performed under visual feed-back. On the other hand, if the animals are trained to perform a complex motor task, the simultaneous cooling of external pallidum and putamen induces the movement disturbances just described but they are not reversed by the intervention of visual feed-back (11). DeLong and Coyle (12) in their experiments of infusion of kainic acid in the internal pallidum of trained monkeys obtained similar results.

b) Substantia nigra

Electrolytic lesions at this level invariably involve both pars compacta and pars reticulata. Unilateral lesions have no obvious motor effects, while bilateral lesions may result in hypokinesia, mild hypotonia and fixed postures (13,14).

Since the two components of the substantia nigra have different functions, the selective lesioning is necessary to understand the contribution of each of them to the observed effects. Till now, there is little or no information about pars reticulata, but the selective destruction of the pars compacta has been achieved by the unilateral injection of 6-hydroxidopamine. This substance produces the extensive destruction of the dopaminergic neurons. In monkeys, the most interesting finding after unilateral injection of 6-hydroxidopamine is, besides hypotonia, appearance of circling behaviour which correlates with asymmetry in striatal dopamine content on the two sides. The short-lasting increase of dopamine due to the degeneration of nigrostriatal pathway terminals of the nigrostriatal pathway is followed by rotation towards the contralateral side. Then the animal enters in a chronic state of deviation towards the side of lesion (15).

Circling is abolished by interruption of nigrostriatal projections, but is not influenced by thalamic and cortical lesions. This implies that the pallido-thalamo-cortical pathway is not responsible for its appearance. On the other hand, experiments of Di Chiara et al. (16) have shown that lesions in the superior colliculus, normally implied in head-eyes orienting behaviours, suppress circling. The results suggest that the nigro-tectal pathway might be responsible for the effect. Recent studies have confirmed this hypothesis (17,18).

c) Subthalamic nucleus

In monkeys, restricted lesions of this nucleus produce a syndrome that closely resembles human hemiballism (19). The involuntary movements appear contralaterally to the lesion and are more prominent in the leg. They may be choreiform, athetoid or ballistic and associated with a variable degree of hypotonia. The same effects can be observed after microinjection in the subthalamic nucleus of GABA-antagonists such as bicuculline (20). Like in man, the involuntary movements may be abolished by the lesion of the contralateral internal pallidum or ventrolateral nucleus of the thalamus (21). This shows that the subthalamic nucleus may normally exert an inhibitory influence on the globus pallidus. As a consequence the appearance of the hyperkinesia might depend on an abnormal pallidal activity (release phenomenon) transmitted, via the thalamus, to the cortex. The recent suggestion that GABA, an inhibitory amino acid, could be the transmitter of the subthalamopallidal projection supports this interpretation (22).

d) Striatum

The striatum constitutes the major input component of the basal ganglia. It receives afferents from different sources, essentially from extensive areas of the neocortex.

Restricted unilateral lesions at this level are without obvious motor effects. On the other hand, if caudate nucleus is largely destroyed, ipsilateral circling behaviour may appear (23).

Bilateral lesions are regularly followed by variable motor abnormalities such as hypertonia and hyperkinesia (24), bilateral inattention, hypokinesia and hyperactive behaviour (25).

Motor effects of lesioning in human subjects affected by movement disorders

The first attempts were inspired by the clinical observation that, after a stroke, the parkinsonian tremor was abolished on the hemiparetic side.

The surgery of the basal ganglia began with the operations of Meyers (26) in parkinsonians. Lesions of globus pallidus are followed by the disappearance of the positive signs of the disease without the draw-back of paresis. However, akinesia remains unchanged.

Other selective stereotaxic lesions, such as in internal pallidum or ventrolateral nuclei of the thalamus, lead to the same results (27,28).

Motor effects of electrical stimulation

Electrical stimulation of the basal ganglia has been performed both in animals and in human subjects during stereotaxic surgery .

a) Animal studies

In monkey, the electrical stimulation of the pallidum induces contraversive head turning and circling (29).

The electrical stimulation of the substantia nigra is also responsible for contraversive head turning and movements of the contralateral limbs. In addition, it induces different behavioural patterns such as licking, chewing and swallowing movements (30).

Similarly, electrical stimulation of the striatum modifies spontaneous motor behaviour and induces contraversive head turning and circling (31), contralateral limbs movements, and " arrest" or "freezing" phenomena (29).

As far as circling behaviour is concerned, the results are in agreement with what has been observed after destruction experiments.

No study of stimulation of the subthalamic nucleus has been performed.

Recent experiments performed in anaesthetized animals have shown that the stimulation of separate zones of striatum and pallidum may differently influence the cortically-induced motor activities. Although inhibitory effects predominate, facilitations have nevertheless been observed (32).

b) Observations in man

The stimulation of the caudate nucleus performed in patients with Parkinson's disease or involuntary movements produces a characteristic arrest of the voluntary activity associated with cessation of speech and contraversive head turning (33).

Electrical stimulation of the pallidum provokes turning of the eyes towards the contralateral side (28). In some cases of athetosis and torsion dystonia, Hassler has reported to have provoked or abolished the abnormal movement on the contralateral side, by varying the frequency of stimulation (28).

Comments

Hemiballism observed after a selective lesion in the subthalamic nucleus, appears as an exception. Other selective unilateral lesions of many parts of the basal ganglia have no apparent effect on untrained monkeys. Only if the lesions are more extensive and bilateral, hypokinesia and/or other so-called extrapyramidal features may appear.

The fact that experimental lesions of striatum are not followed by dyskinesias such as chorea or athetosis like in human disease, suggests that in the latter, the movement abnormalities depend more on the abnormal firing of diseased neurons than on a loss of cells.

On the other hand, experiments with electrical stimulation of various sites of the basal ganglia result in several unspecific effects on motor behaviour such as head turning or flexion movements of the contralateral limbs. The interesting point is that the same movement can be generated by the stimulation of different areas.

The arrest of motricity after striatal stimulation has been observed both in animals and in human subjects.

From all these findings it follows that basal ganglia are implicated both in the regulation of the muscle tone and in production of movements. The exact mechanisms subserving all these functions remain to be elucidated, but it is evident that the basal ganglia have a role more indirect and subtle in the organization of movements than the motor cortex.

It is important to consider that recent studies (34,35) have shown that the efferent pathways of the internal pallidum and of the pars reticulata of the substantia nigra terminate in a portion of the thalamus (VL-VA nuclei) which is not directly connected to the motor cortex, but projects anteriorly to an area (area 6 according to Broadmann) which comprises the premotor area and the supplementary motor area (SMA). From this area, but not from area 4 (motor cortex), Dieckmann and Sasaki (36) were able to record responses after stimulation of the internal pallidum and putamen. The strict relationships of the basal ganglia with the SMA are further supported by the observation that the ablation of this area produces deficits that closely resemble parkinsonism (37). Recent evidence based on both regional blood flow and electrophysiological studies would assign to SMA a role in the preparation of movements. Selective increase of regional blood flow in humans (38) and changes of single neuron activity in monkeys (39) have been recorded from this area when preparing for a complex sequence of movements of the digits performed without sensory guidance. These findings fit well, on the other hand, with the impairment of the self-paced, not visually guided movements observed after cooling of the pallidum (10) (see before) whose projection would reach the SMA. It is then clear that both the basal ganglia and the SMA are essential for movements initiated and executed without exteroceptive guidance, i.e. self-paced, self-guided and spontaneous (40).

SINGLE-CELL RECORDINGS

More recently, the development of techniques of unitary recording has permitted to observe directly the activity of single cells of the basal ganglia (1,41).

a) Spontaneous activity

Spontaneous firing in the different nuclei of the basal ganglia is variable: the neurons of the internal pallidum and of the pars reticulata of the substantia nigra discharge tonically at high frequencies; subthalamic nucleus neurons discharge at a relatively moderate rate; the cells of the pars compacta of the substantia nigra discharge at a low rate. On the contrary most of striatal neurons are silent.

b) Relations to movement

During active movements, many neurons show movement-related changes of activity (41). On the contrary, the pars compacta of the substantia nigra and the caudate nucleus, respectively maintain a tonic activity or keep silent. The temporal relationship between the single unit discharge and the movement is variable. In some neurons the movement-related changes of discharge precede the onset of the correlated EMG activity; however most of pallidal and putaminal neurons discharge after the onset of movement.

This behaviour is somewhat different from that of the motor cortex in which about half of the neurons changes activity before movement. Considering that a large portion of the putaminal afferents comes from the cortex, it is not surprising that discharges in the basal ganglia follow that of the motor cortex cells.

This would imply that basal ganglia are not involved directly in the initiation of movements, but rather in its execution or facilitation. The slowing of movements without changes in reaction times showed in trained monkeys after cooling of internal pallidum supports this view (11). This makes a difference with the motor cortex.

Another interesting aspect emerging from these studies is that in more than half of the responsive neurons, the movement-related changes of activity are not in relation to muscular activity, but depend on other parameters of movement such as its direction or amplitude. These neurons show a directional preference discharging when joint displacement occurs in one direction but not in the other.

Moreover, their firing rate is proportional to the amplitude of movement. The last finding is particularly interesting because it could explain the clinical observation that parkinsonians have difficulty in controlling the amplitude of movements (see below).

c) Somatotopic organization

Single cell recordings have shown that segregated groups of neurons in the putamen, globus pallidus and subthalamic nucleus modulate their activity in relation to movements of specific parts of the body. In other words, in every nucleus, neurons are grouped together in a somatotopic manner. This organization, particularly clear in the putamen (in which clusters of neurons having similar functional properties have been localized), is also found in the other nuclei. These clusters which perhaps constitute the physiological counterpart of the so-called "striosomes", represent the basic functional unit of the striatum much like the functional columns of the neocortex.

This somatotopic arrangement reflects the correspondence with the sensorimotor cortex from which the putamen receives its cortical afferents.

On the other hand, the caudate nucleus does not show somatotopic organization. This nucleus receives afferents from large portions of the neocortex, but not from the sensorimotor areas. Its efferents travel, by a separate route, through the pallidum and ventroanterior nucleus of the thalamus, before reaching the prefrontal areas (42).

From all these findings, some considerations may be drawn:

1) A clear correlation exists between the activity of groups of cells in the basal ganglia and activity in the motor cortex.

2) This correlation is not true for the neurons of the pars compacta of the substantia nigra. Their function is rather one of modulating the striatal function, by releasing dopamine in the striatum.

3) The lack of a tight coupling between neuronal firing in the basal ganglia and specific movements suggests that the basal ganglia play a role somewhat different than cerebellum or motor cortex whose cell-discharge is strictly time-locked to the actual movement.

4) The two constituents of the neostriatum are anatomofunctionally different; a) during movement, putaminal, but not caudate activity is modified. b) the somatotopical organization is absent in the caudate nucleus.

GENERAL VIEW

Complementary anatomical and physiological data suggest that the function of the basal ganglia is intimately related to that of other parts of the brain such as the thalamus and the neocortex. This may explain why some of the signs deriving from their dysfunction appear as due to functional changes in distant structures normally controlled by the basal ganglia activity.

If functional properties and anatomic connections of the basal ganglia are taken into account, it is tempting to consider them as an heterogeneous structure with specialized functions. On these basis, it has been proposed the existence of segregated parallel cortico-subcortical loops subserving motor and complex functions (1,2) (fig.1).

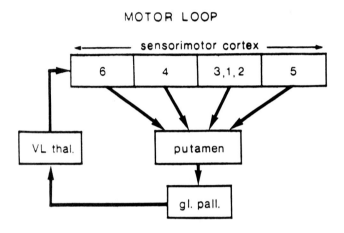

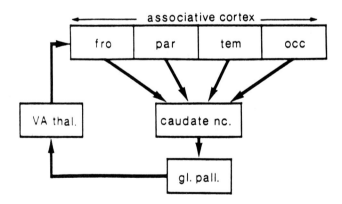

Fig. 1. Basal ganglia loops. Top diagram : numbers refer to Broadmann convention for cortical areas, VL : ventrolateral nucleus. Bottom diagram : Fro : Frontal; Par : parietal; Tem: temporal; occ: occipital; VA : ventroanterior nucleus.

On one side, the motor loop is implicated in the control and execution of motor programmes (see next section); it is constituted by somatotopic projections from the sensorimotor areas directed to the putamen, the pallidum and, via the thalamus back to the cortex, more especially to the SMA (area 6). On the other side, the complex loop is constituted by the diffuse projections from the associative cortex to the caudate nucleus then coming back to the prefrontal cortex via pallidothalamic pathways. This loop might be co-responsible for planning of movements and might implement the function of the higher centers, integrating emotional or motivational drives.

In these loops the striatal neurons discharge after the cortical ones from which they receive the major input. Pallidal cells discharge even later and modulate the thalamus whose activity is directed back to the cortex. In this way, the cortical influences are progressively transformed in spatiotemporal patterns by a process of integration, and multiple influences coming from a large cortical area are reduced into a narrow stream of information.

A third loop involving limbic structures such as the nucleus accumbens could be added to the motor and complex ones. This limbic loop could enable motor actions without the intervention of the cortex. Although the function of this loop is yet poorly known, it is interesting to note that lesions of the nucleus accumbens provoke akinesia (see below).

ASPECTS OF PATHOPHYSIOLOGY

1. Disorders of muscle tone

Rigidity is a "positive" sign of Parkinson's disease. It is characterized by " a constant uniform increase in the resistance to passive movement, throughout the range of joint displacement, while the patient attempts to relax" (43). On the contrary, the muscle tone is generally reduced in the early stage of the classical form of Huntington's chorea. These findings, in agreement with the classical neurophysiological observations (see above), indicate that the basal ganglia play a role in the control of muscle tone. However, as they have no significant direct projections to the spinal cord, this control is necessarily "indirect" and could occur, for example, in motor cortex areas.

Initially, debate concerning pathophysiology of Parkinson's rigidity was centered on the potential role of spinal mechanisms. In the present stage of knowledge, it seems clear that the major spinal mechanisms controlling the stretch reflex excitability, function almost normally (44).

20

An interesting fact relevant to rigidity mechanisms has been reported by Tatton and Lee (45). They have studied the reflex responses evoked by imposed angular joint displacements. They have observed that long-latency responses to stretch (M2-M3) are increased in parkinsonian patients, although M1 response (equivalent to the monosynaptic stretch reflex) remained comparable to that of normal subjects. This increase in M2-M3 responses seems to be correlated with the degree of rigidity (46). To interpret rigidity, it would thus be interesting to know the exact meaning of these responses. Unfortunately, the precise origin of the middle-latency

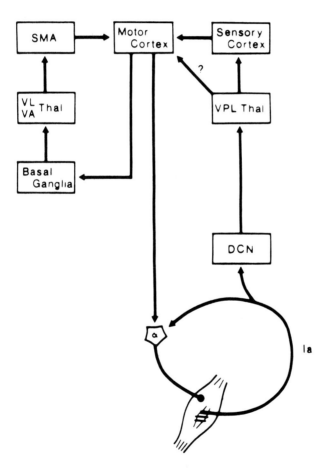

Fig. 2. Tentative diagram of the control, by the basal ganglia of the proprioceptive transcortical loop.
(SMA: supplementary motor area, VL : ventral lateral nucleus, VA : ventral anterior nucleus, VPL : ventral posterior lateral nucleus, DCN : dorsal column nuclei, α : alpha-motoneurons, Ia : Ia afferent fibers.

component (M2) of the stretch reflex remains still debated (for review, see ref. 47, 48, 49, 50). It has been postulated that the middle-latency response (M2) is mediated, at least partially, by a transcortical pathway involving the motor cortex (51, 52, 53). As a consequence, rigidity could be the result of an hyperexcitability in transcortical loops, normally inhibited by basal ganglia function, directly or indirectly.

This is in agreement with studies in animal models of parkinsonian rigidity (54) and with human data obtained after neurosurgical procedures: relief of rigidity is obtained after lesioning of either the globus pallidus or the ventrolateral nucleus of the thalamus (1). This view is also supported by the opposite results recently obtained in hypotonic patients by Noth et al. (55). These authors have in fact shown that the long-latency EMG responses are selectively decreased or absent in patients with Huntington's chorea.

Although the precise mode of control is not yet clear, a diagram explaning the possible role exerted by the basal ganglia on the transcortical stretch reflex gain, is presented in fig. 2.

2. Disorders of voluntary movement

Parkinson's disease is regarded as the best human model of basal ganglia motor dysfunction. However, it is well known that Parkinson's disease involves structures other than the basal ganglia (56). Although it is not a perfect model, Parkinson's disease has been largely studied to elucidate motor functions of the basal ganglia. Parkinson's disease is generally accompanied by akinesia defined as "a disorder characterized by poverty and slowness of initiation and execution of willed and associated movements and difficulty in changing one motor pattern to another, in the absence of paralysis. The term of bradykinesia should be reserved for slowness in the execution of movement" (43). It is important to emphasize that akinesia is not secondary to rigidity or to a general inhibition of motoneurones, but must be regarded as a primary defect in motor organization in Parkinson's disease.

Several behavioural studies have been performed in order to analyze the specific motor disorder of Parkinson's Disease. At this stage, it is relevant to summarize briefly the normal sequence of processes involved in voluntary movement. Execution of voluntary movement requires two main steps (for review, see ref. 57, 58, 59, 3).

1. formation and assembly of the motor plan
2. initiation and execution of the motor plan

1. The motor planning

After the perceptual process ("idea to move"), the appropriate motor response has to be formulated. This requires firstly the selection of subroutines (motor programmes) and then, their assembly into appropriate sequences in order to build up the motor plan. Programming and planning involve basically basal ganglia, cerebellar hemispheres and associative cortex (58).

2. Its execution

Once correctly formulated the motor plan must be executed and the motor commands transferred to motor cortex before descending to the spinal motoneurons. This requires the initiation of the motor plan and the sequential switching from one motor programme to another. The execution of the motor plan involves the motor cortex, the pyramidal tract, the motoneurons and the skeletal muscles but also the reafferences (joint, muscles etc) coming back to the CNS.

On the basis of this simplified scheme of movement organization, one can question which step of this process is disturbed in akinesia.

A number of studies, based on the reaction-time paradigm, have assessed the ability of Parkinsonians to program the appropriate motor response. Although it is well known that simple reaction-time is increased in Parkinson's disease, the difference between simple and choice reaction-time has been shown to be in the normal range (60). This difference, called "the central delay", is regarded as the time to select the appropriate motor program. It can thus be concluded that programming is normal in Parkinson's disease, at least for simple tasks. Other evidence suggests that parkinsonian patients are able to prepare for motor action in a normal fashion : Heilman (61) for example found that Parkinsonians are still able to improve reaction time in the same range as normal subjects when a warning signal is given 0.5 or 1 sec before the cue. From this observation, Marsden (62) concludes that patients with Parkinson's disease can "select an appropriate motor program, in advance of the stimulus to move ". Nevertheless, this conclusion remains still open to discussions. Flowers (63,64) observed that patients with parkinsonism are less successful in employing predictive motor acts. These patients do not perform correctly a ballistic movement; this latter, being preprogrammed, requires the intervention of a predictive factor; parkinsonians fail to reach the target at once and the resulting movement is hypometric. Moreover, Parkinsonians are more dependent on visual feedback than normal subjects to reach a target (65). From these data, Marsden (62) concludes that patient with

Parkinson's disease can :

1. correctly perceive stimulus (to move)

2. take appropriate action by selecting the correct motor programme

3. but are less successful in employing predictive motor action and are more dependent on the visual feedback.

In the light of these observations, akinesia might not be attributed to a defect of motor programming. However, even if the motor response is correctly programmed, it is not sure that the programme reachs the motor cortex normally. To answer this question, Kornhuber and Deecke (66) have recorded the premovement potential (Bereitschaftspotential or readiness potential - RP) occuring about 1 sec before the onset of movement. This RP is believed to originate from the motor and premotor cortex. In Parkinson's disease, it was found that RP over the pre-rolandic cortex is clearly reduced whereas it remains normal over the vertex.At that site, the generator is probably the supplementary motor area (SMA) (67,68). From these data, the RP amplitude decrease could be attributed to a deficit in the transfer of the motor programme from the basal ganglia, via premotor cortex to motor cortex. This hypothesis is supported by the fact that whereas the correct muscle is selected and the reciprocal inhibition between agonist and antagonist muscles is preserved, the amplitude of the first agonist burst is reduced and movement undershoots the target (69). As a result, a serie of small agonist burst is necessary to reach the target. Similar hypometric movements have been described in ocular saccades. The overall conclusion from these data is that in patients with Parkinson's disease the content of motor programmes is either specified incorrectly or does not reach the motor cortex normally.

So far, only simple movements have been considered, but it is well known from clinical observations that patient with Parkinson's disease have difficulties in executing repetitive, concurrent or sequential movements. According to Marsden (3,62), the critical feature in Parkinson's disease is the inability to execute learned motor plan and to switch from one motor programme to another. "Freezing", that may be exemplified in speech, handwriting and walking, illustrates this defect. As a consequence, "there is a fundamental breakdown in the capacity to run the sequence of movements, that composes motor plan. In other words, the sequence of motor plan does not run smoothly in Parkinson's disease " (70).

This suggestion leads to the hypothesis that the basal ganglia play a role in running, automatically, the sequence of motor programmes included in the motor plan. From these behavioural motor studies, the Parkinsonian motor deficit can be equated to an inability to specify correctly the content of motor programmes and to run their sequence automatically, switching from one programme to another.

Pathophysiological and biochemical approaches to the neural basis of akinesia have been essentially directed to the nigrostriatal,dopaminergic fibers. In the experimental animal, akinesia results from bilateral destruction of ascending dopaminergic pathways or from the administration of drugs that block synthesis of dopamine or prevent its storage (reserpine). A specific role for the nucleus accumbens - which receives dopaminergic fibers from the ventral tegmental area (VTA) -is suggested by the experimental finding that an increase of spontaneous movements occurs following injection of dopamine in this nucleus. Similarly, injection of dopamine into the nucleus accumbens counteracts akinesia but not rigidity in reserpine-induced parkinsonism. On the other hand, its injection into the striatum abolishes rigidity without alleviating akinesia. These experimental observations have been confirmed by the finding that the concentration of dopamine in nucleus accumbens of Parkinsonians is markedly reduced (71). Thus the impairment of mesolimbic (VTA-accumbens) dopaminergic pathway might be one of the factors in the pathogenesis of akinesia.

REFERENCES
1. De Long MR, Georgopoulos AP (1981) Motor functions of the basal ganglia. In: Brooks VB (ed) Handbook of Physiol. Section I, vol. II, Amer. Physiol. Society, Bethesda, pp 1017-1061.

2. Brooks VB (1986) The neural basis of motor control. Oxford Univ. Press, Oxford, 330pp

3. Marsden CD (1982) The mysterious motor function of the basal ganglia : the Robert Wartenberg lecture. Neurology 32: 514-539.

4. Delwaide PJ, Gonce M (in press) Pathophysiology of Parkinson's signs. In: J Jankovic, E. Tolosa (eds), Parkinson's Disease and other movement disorders,Urban and Schwarzenberg, Medical Publishers.

5. Damasio AR (1985) Language and the basal ganglia. In EV Evarts, SP Wise, D Bousfield (eds). The motor system in neurobiology. Elsevier, Amsterdam, pp 288-291.

6. Wilson SA (1914) An experimental research into the anatomy and physiology of the corpus striatum. Brain 36: 427-492.

7. Kennard MA (1944) Experimental analysis of the functions of the basal ganglia in monkeys and chimpanzees. J. Neurophysiol. 7: 127-148.

8. Laursen AM (1955) An experimental study of the pathways from the basal ganglia. J. Comp. Neurol. 102: 1-25.

9. Denny-Brown D (1962) The basal ganglia and their relation to disorders of movement. Oxford Univ. Press, London.

10. Hore J, Meyer-Lohmann J, Brooks VB (1977) Basal ganglia cooling disables learned arm movements of monkeys in the absence of visual guidance. Science 195: 585-586.

11. Hore J, Vilis T (1980) Arm movement performance during reversible basal ganglia lesions in the monkey. Exp. Brain Res 39: 217-228.

12. De Long MR, Coyle JT (1979) Globus pallidus lesions in the monkey produced by kainic acid: histologic and behavioural effects. Appl. Neurophysiol. 42: 95-97.

13. Carpenter MB, Mc Masters RE (1964) Lesions of the substantia nigra in the rhesus monkey. Efferent fiber degeneration and behavioural observations. Am. J. Anat. 114: 293-320.

14. Stern G (1960) The effects of lesions in the substantia nigra. Brain 89: 449-478.

15. Jungberg TI, Ungerstedt U (1976) Sensory inattention produced by 6-hydroxydopamine-induced degeneration of ascending dopamine neurons. Exp. Neurol. 53: 585-600.

16. Di Chiara G, Morelli M, Imperato A, Porceddu ML (1982) A reevaluation of the role of superior colliculus in turning behaviour. Brain Res. 237: 61-77

17. Hikosaka O, Wurtz RH (1983) Visual and oculomotor functions of monkey substantia nigra pars reticulata. Relations of substantia nigra to superior colliculus. J. Neurophysiol; 49: 1285-1301

18. Chevalier G, Vacher S, Denian JM (1984) Inhibitory nigral influence on tecto-spinal neurons. A possible implication of basal ganglia in orienting behaviour. Exp. Brain Res. 53: 320-326.

19. Carpenter MB, Whittier JR, Mettler FA (1950) Analysis of choreoid hyperkinesia in the rhesus monkey. Surgical and pharmacological analysis of hyperkinesia resulting from lesions of the subthalamic nucleus of Luys. J. Comp. Neurol. 92: 293-331.

20. Crossman AR, Sambrook MA, Jackson A (1984) Experimental hemichorea/hemiballismus in the monkey. Brain 107: 579-596.

21. Martin JP, Mc Coul IR (1959) Acute hemiballismus treated by ventrolateral thalamolysis. Brain 82: 104-108.

22. Nauta HJ, Cuenod M (1982) Perikaryal cell labeling in the subthalamic nucleus following the injection of (3H)-8-aminobutyric acid into the pallidal complex : an autoradiographic study in cat. Neuroscience 7: 2725-2734.

23. Mettler FA, Mettler CC (1942) The effects of striatal injury. Brain 65: 242-255.

24. Liddell EG, Phillips CG (1940) Experimental lesions in the basal ganglia of the cat. Brain 63: 264-274.

25. Villablanca JR, Marcus RJ, Olmstead CE (1976) Effects of caudate nuclei or frontal cortical ablations in cats. I. Neurology and gross behaviour. Exp. Neurol. 52: 389-420.

26. Meyers R (1942) The modification of alternating tremors, rigidity and festination of surgery of the basal ganglia. Res. Publ. Assoc. Res. Nerv. Ment. Dis. 21: 602-665.

27. Spiegel EA, Wycis HT, Freed H (1952) Stereoencephalotomy, thalotomy and related procedures. J. Am. Med. Assoc. 148: 446-451.

28. Hassler R, Reichert T, Mundinger F, Umbach W, Ganlberger JA (1960) Physiological observations in stereotaxic operations in extrapyramidal motor disturbances. Brain 83: 337-350

29. Buchwald NA, Ervin FR (1957) Evoked potentials and behaviour. A study of responses to subcortical stimulation in the awake, unrestrained animal. Electroenceph. Clin. Neurophysiol. 9: 477-496.

30. York DH (1973) Motor responses induced by stimulation of the substantia nigra. Exp. Neurol. 41: 321-330.

31. Kitsikis A, Rougel A (1968) The effect of caudate stimulation on conditioned motor behaviour in monkeys. Physiol. Behav. 3: 831-837.

32. Newton RA, Price DD (1975) Modulation of cortical and pyramidal tract induced motor responses by electrical stimulation of the basal ganglia. Brain Res. 85: 403-422.

33. Van Burin JM, Li CL, Oyemann GA (1966) The frontostriatal arrest response in man. Electroenceph. Clin. Neurophysiol; 21: 114-130.

34. Carpenter MB (1981) Anatomy of the corpus striatum and brainstem integrating systems. In : Brooks VB (ed), Handbook of Physiol. Section I, vol. II, Motor Control. Amer. Physiol. Soc, pp 947-995

35. Tracey DJ, Asanuma C, Jones EG, Porter R (1980) Thalamic relay to motor cortex; afferent pathways from brain stem, cerebellum and spinal cord in monkeys. J. Neurophysiol. 44: 532-554.

36. Dieckmann G, Sasaki K (1970) Recruiting responses in the cerebral cortex produced by putamen and pallidum stimulation. Exp. Brain Res 10: 236-250.

37. Boetz MI (1974) Frontal lobe tumors. In : Vinken PJ, Bruyn GW (eds), Handbook of Clinical Neurology, Elsevier, Amsterdam, 234-280.

38. Roland PE, Larsen B, Lassen NA, Skinhoj E (1980) Supplementary motor area and other cortical areas in organization of voluntary movements in man. J. Neurophysiol. 43: 118-136.

39. Tanji J, Taniguchi K, Saga T (1980) Supplementary motor area : neural response to motor instructions. J. Neurophysiol. 43: 60-68.

40. Evarts EV, Wise SP (1984) Basal ganglia outputs and motor control. In Function of the basal ganglia, Pitman, London, pp 83-102.

41. DeLong MR, Georgopoulos AP, Crutcher MD, Mitchell SJ, Richardson RT, Alexander GE (1984) Functional organization of the basal ganglia: contributions of single-cell recording studies. In: Functions of the basal ganglia. Pitman, London, Ciba Foundation Symposium 107, PP 64-82.

42. Kievit J, Kuypers GJ (1977) organization of the thalamo-cortical connections to the frontal lobe in the rhesus monkey. Exp. Brain Res. 29: 299-322.

43. Lakke PW (1981) Classification of extrapyramidal disorders. J. Neurol. Sci. 51:311-327.

44. Delwaide PJ (1985) Are there modifications in spinal cord functions of parkinsonian patients ? In: PJ Delwaide, A Agnoli (eds) Clinical Neurophysiology in Parkinsonism. Elsevier, Amsterdam, pp 19-32.

45. Tatton WG, Lee RG (1975) Evidence for abnormal long-loop reflexes in rigid Parkinsonian patients. Brain Res. 96:108-113.

46. Mortimer JA, Webster DD (1978) Relationships between quantitative measures of rigidity and tremor and the electromyographic responses to load perturbations in unselected normal subjects and Parkinson patients. In: JE Desmedt (ed), Cerebral motor control in man : long-loop mechanisms. Karger, Basel, pp 342-360.

47. Wiesendanger M, Miles TS (1982) Ascending pathway of low-threshold muscle afferents to the cerebral cortex and its possible role in motor control. Physiol. Rev. 62: 1234-1270.

48. Hagbarth KE, Hagglund JV, Wallin EV, Young RR (1981) Grouped spindle and electromyographic responses to abrupt wrist extension movements in man. J. Physiol. (Lobd) 312:81-96.

49. Tatton WG, Bedingham W, Verrier MC, Bruce IC, Blair RD (1984) Abnormalities of mechanoreceptor-evoked electromyographic activity in central motor disorders. In: Struppler A, Weindl A (Eds), Electromyography and Evoked Potentials - Theories and applications. Springer-Verlag, pp 9-18

50.Matthews PB (1986) What are the afferents of origin of the human stretch reflex, and is it a purely spinal reaction ? In: Freund HJ, Buttner U, Cohen B, Noth J (Eds), Progress in Brain Research, vol. 64, Elsevier, Amsterdam, pp 55-66.

51.Phillips CG (1969) The Ferrier Lecture 1968. Motor apparatus of the baboon's hand. Proc. R. Soc. London B 173: 141-174.

52.Marsden CD, Merton PA, Morton HB (1973) Is the human stretch reflex cortical rather than spinal ? Lancet 1:759-761.

53.Cheney PD, Fetz EE (1984) Corticomotoneuronal cells contribute to long-latency stretch reflexes in the Rhesus monkey.J. Physiol (Lond) 349:249-272.

54.Tatton WG, Eastman MJ, Bedingham W, Verrier MC, Bruce IC (1984) Defective utilization of sensory input as the basis for bradykinesia, rigidity and decreased movement repertoire in Parkinson's disease : a hypothesis. Can J. Neurol. Sci. 11: 136-143.

55.Noth J, Friedemann HH, Podoll K, Lange HW (1983) Absence of long-latency reflexes to imposed finger displacements in patients with Huntington's disease. Neurosci. Lett. 35: 97-100.

56.Marsden CD (1984) Function of the basal ganglia as revealed by cognitive and motor disorders in Parkinson's disease. Can. J. Neurol. Sci. 11: 129-135.

57.Allen GI, Tsukahara N (1974) Cerebrocerebellar communication systems. Physiol. Rev. 54: 957-1006.

58.Brooks VB (1979) Motor programs revisited. In: Talbott RE, Humphrey DR (eds), Posture and movement. Raven Press, New York, pp 13-49.

59.Paillard J (1982) Apraxia and the neurophysiology of motor control. Phil. Trans. R. Soc. Lond. B298, pp 111-134.

60.Evarts EV, Teravainen M, Calne DB (1981) Reaction time in Parkinson's disease. Brain 104: 167-186.

61.Heilman KM, Bowers D, Watson RT, Greer M (1976) Reaction times in Parkinson's disease. Arch. Neurol. 33:139-140.

62.Marsden CD (1985) Defects of movement in Parkinson's disease. In: PJ Delwaide, A Agnoli (eds), Clinical Neurophysiology in Parkinsonism, Elsevier, Amsterdam, pp 107-115.

63.Flowers KA (1976) Visual "closed-loop" and "open-loop" characteristics of voluntary movement in patients with parkinsonism and intention tremor. Brain 99: 269-310.

64.Flowers KA (1978) Lack of prediction in the motor behaviour of parkinsonism. Brain 104: 35-52.

65.Stern Y, Mayeux R, Rosen J, Ilson J (1983) Perceptual motor dysfunction in Parkinson's disease : a deficit in sequential and predictive voluntary movement. J. Neurol. Neurosurg. Psychiat. 46: 145-151.

66.Kornhuber HH, Deecke L (1965) Hirnpotentialänderungen bei Willkürbewegungen und passiven Bewegungen des Menschen: Bereitschaftpotential und reafferente Potentiale. Pflügers Arch. 284: 1-17.

67.Shibasaki M, Shima F, Kuroiwa Y (1978) Clinical studies of the movement-related cortical potential (MP) and the relationship between the dentato rubro-thalamic pathway and readiness potential (RP) J. Neurol; 219: 15-25.

68.Deecke L (1985) Cerebral potentials related to voluntary actions: parkinsonian and normal subjects. In: PJ Delwaide, A Agnoli (eds), Clinical Neurophysiology in Parkinsonism. Elsevier, Amsterdam, pp 91-105.

69.Hallett M, Khoshbin S (1980) A physiological mechanism of bradykinesia. Brain 103:301-304.

70.Barbeau A (1973) Biology of the striatum. In GE Gaull (ed), Biology of brain dysfunction, pp 333-350.

71.Price KS, Farley IJ, Hornykiewicz O (1978) Neurochemistry of Parkinson's disease:relation between striatal and limbic dopamine. Adv. Biochem; Psychopharmacol. 19: 293-300.

© 1987 Elsevier Science Publishers B.V. (Biomedical Division)
Extrapyramidal disorders in childhood
L. Angelini et al. editors

EXTRAPYRAMIDAL DISORDERS IN CHILDHOOD

NICOLO' RIZZUTO, ALESSANDRO SALVIATI, TIZIANA CAVALLARO
Cattedra di Neuropatologia, Istituto di Neurologia, Universita' di
Verona, 37134 Verona (Italia)

INTRODUCTION

A number of heterogeneous mechanisms may produce dystonic-dyskinetic syndromes in childhood. Most frequently the cause, e.g. perinatal hypoxia-ischemia, produces lesions of a developing or a normally
developed nervous structure, at a defined time. The resulting syndrome shows static, non-progressive, clinical characteristics. On
the other hand, the pathogenetic mechanism may act discretely for a
long period of time, e.g. metabolic disorders, or "degenerative"
conditions producing slow and continuous death of neuronal elements;
slowly progressive course will characterize the latter clinical
syndromes.

NON-PROGRESSIVE DISORDERS
Extrapyramidal Cerebral Palsy
  Perinatal Causes. Cerebral palsy is classified into two major
groups: spastic (pyramidal) and extrapyramidal (choreoathetoid).
Approximately 15% of cases of cerebral palsy are classified as
extrapyramidal (Marquis et al, 1982).
  Kernicterus (bilirubin enchephalopathy) has been, until 20 years
ago, a major cause of extrapyramidal cerebral palsy. Full term or
pre-term neonate low activity of liver uridin diphosphoglucuronyl
transferase results in inadequate capacity to conjugate the overload
of bilirubin after haemolysis in cases of blood group Rh or ABO
incompatibility. A low blood albumin level (frequent in premature
infants) and/or acidosis are additional negative factors. The mechanisms by which unconjugated bilirubin crosses the blood-brain
barrier is not fully understood. Hypoxic damage is supposed to be a
major cause (Lucey et al, 1964). Pathologically liquor, meninges,
cerebellum, parahippocampal gyrus and basal ganglia are yellow
stained. Kernicterus corresponds to the acute phase of the disease;
after the first postnatal week the yellow staining disappears.
Later, neuronal loss and fibrillary gliosis are observed.
  Due to the available prophylactic measures, Kernicterus virtually
disappeared as a cause of brain damage and has been replaced by
perinatal hypoxia-ischemia as a major cause of extrapyramidal cerebral palsy. Since anoxic insults cause diffuse damage of the nervous
system, mental retardation and epilepsy are often associated. The
pathological sequelae of hypoxic-ischemic damage are varied. Multi-
cystic structures can be present in various degrees until "honey-
comb" appearence. Ulegyria and gyral scarring are due to segmental
neuronal loss. Cortical laminar or nodular atrophy is a frequent
finding. Intracerebral, subependymal or intraventricular haemorrhage
can be present. In the basal ganglia, status marmoratus can be

observed. The latter pathological entity, often associated with cortical lesions, is characterized by bilateral whitish spots or streaks, resembling the pattern of marble, in corpus striatum and, less frequently, in caudate and thalamic nuclei. On microscopic examination, focal loss of neurons, glial scarring, bundles of abnormally distributed myelinated fibers, encrusted or ferruginated neurons are typical findings (Borit and Herndon, 1970).

Postnatal Causes. Cyanotic heart disease: hypoxiemia determines neuronal necrosis. Thrombosis and embolia, frequently after heart surgery, cause various brain lesions, such as leucomalacia and infarcts. Hypoglycemia: small-for-date infants frequently show inadequate regulation of blood glycemic levels, with resulting hypoglycemia. The pathology (neuronal necrosis) is similar to that of hypoxic-ischemic states (Larroche, 1984). Head injury: focal damage can result from cerebral contusion, intracranial and/or intracerebral hematomas, traumatic thrombosis, axonal injury and fat embolism. Diffuse damage can be produced by brain oedema.

Acute-chronic intoxication. CO gives rise to anaemic hypoxia. Symmetrical circumscribed macroscopic infarcts are often seen in globus pallidus, hippocampus and substantia nigra (zona reticularis). Neuroleptic drugs: respiratory and/or cardiac failure can occur during severe intoxication; the resulting hypoxic-ischaemic state is cause of the brain damage. Lead: chronic lead intoxication produces encephalopathy by primary damage to vascular endothelium. Symmetrical pallidal necrosis and diffuse cerebral lesions can occur. Acute intoxication frequently determines, by the same pathogenetic mechanism, brain oedema of various severity (Jacobs and Le Quesne, 1984).Viral encephalitis: Acute infectious encephalitis is characterized by infection and destruction of neurons and glial cells. Glial scarring develop in survivors. Acute postinfectious encephalitis may complicate measles, chickenpox, rubella and mumps; lympho-monocytic perivascular cuffing and demyelination suggest an immunological pathogenesis.

PROGRESSIVE DISORDERS
Junenile Parkinsonism
Juvenile Parkinsonism, defined as parkinsonism manifesting clinically below 40 years of age, affects about 10% of the whole parkinsonian population (Narabayashi et al.,1986); in 1% of the patients the symptoms start between 10 and 20 years of age (Martin et al.,1973 a,b).

Clinical picture is characterized by rigidity, tremor and akinesia in a slowly progressive course. Difficulty of gait and muscle stiffness are usually the first signs. Dystonic signs of the legs and dystonic postures of the trunk are often present. In general, tremor at rest is rare. The symptoms are usually bilateral from the beginning, unlikely classical Parkinson disease. The slow progression and the good response to levodopa therapy make the patients able to continue work and social activity for longer periods than classical Parkinson disease patients. However, severe adverse effects to therapy have been described. Mental changes, tendency to develop depressive states, autonomic dysfunction are neither marked nor frequent.

Early onset Parkinson patients have affected relatives in higher percentages than classic idiopathic Parkinson patients, suggesting that genetic background might be an important etiological factor (Narabayashi et al, 1986).

Neuropathological changes are similar to those observed in classic idiopathic Parkinson disease: loss of pigmented cells in substantia nigra (zona compacta) and in locus coeruleus; corresponding gliosis; inclusion bodies of Lewy type. The latter finding consists of concentric hyalin cytoplasmic inclusions, formed by filaments, loosely packed in the outer zone, densely packed and mixed with granular material in the central core; they are recognized by anti-filaments antibodies in immunohistochemistry (Kahn et al, 1985).

Juvenile Huntington's Chorea

This is a progressive hereditary (autosomal dominant) disease, characterized by a movement disorder (usually chorea), dementia and psychiatric changes. A number of cases have been described with onset below 20 years of age. Typically, the patient's affected parent is almost always the father (Bruyn and Went, 1986). Gait abnormalities, with frequent falls, slight personality changes and gradual withdrawal of contact with environment are the first insidious changes after a normal development. The disease may show a choreatic or hypokinetic-rigid evolution, or a mixture of dystonic and hypokinetic symptoms. Rigidity and hypokinesia are, however, much more frequent than in adult-onset forms. Cerebellar signs (ataxia, dys/adiadochokinesis) are present in 50% of cases. Dementia is rapid and severe. Epilepsy (absences, grand mal attacks, status epilepticus) is an important feature in 40% of cases. The course is rapid (2-6 years) (Stevens, 1973).

Neuropathological examination reveals a moderate cerebral atrophy, severe atrophy of the corpus striatum, and of cerebellum. On microscopic examination, severe loss of neurons in the caudate nucleus and putamen, usually with relative sparing of the large neurons, is observed; reactive astrogliosis is present in the same areas. Globus pallidus, thalamus, substantia nigra (zona reticularis) are also affected in a variable degree. Loss of Purkinje and dentate nucleus cells is severe in juvenile cases.

The cause is unknown and the theraphy is symptomatic.

The gene responsible for the disease has been localized to the short arm of the chromosome 4 (Gusella et al., 1983) by a linked DNA restriction fragment lenght polymorphism; it is associated with four different patterns of DNA fragments (haplotypes) which are present in varying frequencies in the normal population. These haplotypes have predictive value in presymptomatic individuals, when one or both parent's genotype can be examined, since the frequency of genetic recombination between the restriction fragments and the Huntington's chorea gene is very low.

Olivo-Ponto-Cerebellar Atrophy

The typical signs and symptoms are progressive cerebellar ataxia of the trunk and limbs, impairment of equilibrium and gait, scanning speech and nystagmus. There is usually a familial distribution; sporadic cases have been described.

Pathologically, there is atrophy of the ventral part of pons, of the middle cerebellar peduncles and of inferior olives. Almost complete loss of myelin staining of the transverse fibers of the pons, loss of neurons of inferior olives and of olivo-cerebellar fibers, loss of Purkinje cells with relative sparing of vermis and flocculus are the main pathological features.

Extrapyramidal symptoms (rigidity, immobile facies, and parkinsonian tremor), together with ophthalmoplegia and dementia, are sometimes present.These cases show, in addition to the olivo-ponto-cerebellar degeneration, loss of neurons, with fibrous gliosis, in striatum (expecially putamen) and substantia nigra. According to Konysmark and Weiner classification of olivo-ponto-cerebellar atrophy (1970), these cases belong either to type 2 (recessive inheritance) or to type 5 (dominant inheritance).

Neuro-axonal Dystrophies

Neuroaxonal dystrophy is defined as a peculiar swelling of the axon containing tubular structures, neurofilaments, vesicles, masses of smooth membranes and mitochondria. These changes can be found in healthy individuals, with a frequency steadily increasing with age, in the nuclei of the posterior columns of the lower medulla, in the substantia nigra (zona reticularis), and in the globus pallidus (medial part). Their pathogenesis has not been clarified; however, a defect in axonal transport governing the turnaround mechanisms between anterograde and retrograde transport is suspected.

In primary neuroaxonal dystrophy diseases, this age-related phenomenon is abnormally enhanced in quantity and intensity, showing wider distribution (Seitelberger, 1986).

NEUROAXONAL DISTROPHIES

Hallervorden-Spatz Disease
Infantile Neuroaxonal Dystrophy
Late Infantile - Juvenile Neuroaxonal Dystrophy
Neuroaxonal Leukodystrophy

Hallervorden-Spatz Disease

The condition, in many cases presenting an autosomal recessive inheritance, is clinically characterized by progressive rigidity, often associated with choreic or athetoid movements or torsion dystonia, in most cases beginning in the first or second decade. Mental deterioration and epileptic convulsions may be present. A "frozen", painful, expression with risus sardonicus is frequently seen. Reflexes are hyperactive. Ataxia, tremor, nystagmus and facial grimacing are seen in some patients. Three types are recognized according to the age of onset: late infantile (3 months to 6 years), classic (7 to 15 years) and adult or late (22 to 64 years) (Jellinger, 1973).

Pathologically, a rust-brown discoloration of the globus pallidus and substantia nigra (zona reticularis) due to pigment accumulation, is macroscopically seen. Strongly siderophilic incrustations of the small vessels and free-lying mulberry concretions (pseudocalcium) are also present. Axonal spheroids are frequent, expecially in the pallidum, substantia nigra (zona reticularis), subthalamic nucleus, tegmentum of the medulla, cerebral cortex and spinal cord. Loss of nerve cells with fibrous gliosis is seen in these areas and also in the striatum and cerebellar cortex. An enzymatic block of the metabolic pathway from cysteine to taurine has been proposed as the pathogenetic mechanism (Perry et al, 1985). Definite diagnosis requires autopsy.

Infantile Neuroaxonal Dystrophy

Described by Seitelberger (1952), this disease is trasmitted as an autosomal recessive trait, affecting all races and both sexes. Psychomotor retardation begins within the second year of age. Muscular hypotonia and areflexia, followed by spasticity and/or rigidity are often observed. Cerebellar symptoms, blindness with optic atrophy, strabismus, deafness, impairment of vestibular function, hyperesthesia, dysautonomia usually develop. Convulsions may occur; mental deterioration steadily develops. Most of the patients die before age 6.

Neuropathological examination reveals cerebral and cerebellar atrophy. No pigmentation is detected in globus pallidus and substantia nigra. The presence of axonal spoheroids is the prominent feature, mostly in brain stem, dorsal horns of the spinal cord, cerebellar cortex, substantia nigra, putamen, pallidus and thalamus. Sensory and motor peripheral nerve terminals are also affected. Long tract degeneration is often present. Status dysmyelinatus of the globus pallidus is a characteristic finding. Loss of nerve cells with reactive astrocytic gliosis is observed in the affected areas. Nerve, muscle, rectal or conjunctival biopsy is confirmatory when spheroids are found in nerve or at the neuromuscular junction. However, since the axonal spheroids can be a rare feature, normal peripheral nerve or even cortical biopsy does not rule out the diagnosis. The genetic/biochemical basis of the disease is unknown.

Late Infantile and Juvenile Neuroaxonal Dystrophy

This group is defined by an onset after 2 years of age, with progressive rigidity and spasticity, cerebellar dysfunction, speech and visual deterioration, dementia and convulsions. Autosomic recessive and sporadic cases have been reported. Numerous large axonal spheroids are widespread through the grey matter (status globosus), sometimes producing an increase in volume of the affected nuclei (pseudohypertrophy). Degeneration and degradation of the spheroids can produce spongiosis or even cystic appearence of the grey matter. Iron and brown glial pigments can be detected in the pallidonigral system.

Other neuropathological findings can be associated in a number of cases: degeneration of pyramidal tracts and motor neuron atrophy, Lewy-body inclusions, Rosenthal fibers, lipid storage disorder (Seitelberger, 1986).

Neuroaxonal Leukodystrophy

This entity is defined by the presence of numerous axonal swellings mainly affecting the white matter, producing widespread demyelination in cerebral and cerebellar hemispheres, with partial preservation of subcortical fibers. Leukodystrophy is supposed to be secondary to the axonal spheroids formation (Seitelberger, 1986).

Pallidal Degenerations

The globus pallidus can be selectively affected by degenerative changes (pure efferent pallidal system degeneration) or by variable combinations of simultaneous neural degeneration. Loss of neurons and of nerve fibers and demyelination of specific neural pathways are the neuropathological hallmarks. These forms are rare; both familial (autosomic recessive) and sporadic cases have been reported.

Pure pallidal atrophy. In these very rare cases, choreoathetotic hyperkinesia gradually evolving to a final rigid-akinetic state, torsion dystonia without mental deterioration were clinically observed. Symmetrical degeneration of the globus pallidus with fibrillary gliosis, demyelination of the ansa lenticularis and pallidoluysian tract were found. The other nuclei were spared, showing only increased lipofuscin content (van Bogaert, 1946).

Pure pallidoluyisan atrophy. Torticollis and a complex athetotic-parkinsonian syndrome respectively were clinically observed in two families. Bilateral symmetrical loss of neurons, demyelination and fibrillary gliosis in the globus pallidus, subthalamic nucleus and ansa lenticularis were the characteristic post-mortem findings (van Bogaert, 1941).

In pallido nigral (McCormick and Lemmi, 1965) and pallido-luysio-nigral-atrophy (Contamin et al, 1971), progressive akinesia and dystonic rigidity without tremor were the characteristic clinical features. Neuropathological examination revealed symmetrical atrophy with gliosis of the globus pallidus, subthalamic nucleus, substantia nigra, demyelination of the ansa and fasciculus lenticularis. Mild astrocytosis was observed in otherwise intact thalamus and brainstem tegmentum.

Dentato-rubro-pallido-luysian atrophy (Titela and van Bogaert, 1946). In this form, probably inherited as autosomal recessive trait, cerebellar efferent pathway (dentato-rubral) and the pallido-luysian fibers degenerate simultaneously. These cases, in which ataxia and choreoathetosis coexist, are classified by Iizuka et al

(1984) in three types:

a) ataxo-choreoathetoid type, in which cerebellar symptoms are succeeded by extrapyramidal symptoms;

b) pseudo-Huntington type, in which slight cerebellar signs are soon covered by choreic movements, with severe mental changes;

c) myoclonus epilepsy type, with myoclonus, epileptic seizures, ataxia, dysarthria, dementia.

Dentate nucleus shows constantly a severe loss of neurons with dense gliosis. Pallidus (especially the outer segment), subthalamic and red nucleus are constantly involved with variable degree of degenerative changes. Demyelination and atrophy of the brainstem tegmentum, inferior cerebellar peduncle, spino-cerebellar tract and posterior column of the spinal cord may be associated in various degrees and combinations.

NEUROMETABOLIC DISORDERS

Information regarding biochemical defects in neurological disorders is continuously increasing. Many of them produce generalized effects involving all the cellular components of the nervous system, together with other organs and systems (e.g. disorders of aminoacid metabolism, glycogenoses). Many of them produce dystonic-dyskinetic abnormalities. Some affect specific neural constituents with a diffuse involvement (e.g. leukodystrophies). Other defects produce alterations affecting, at least at the beginning, a few specific neuronal systems, mimiking the progressive selective damage of degenerative disease (e.g. malic enzyme deficiency in spino-cerebellar ataxia, dystonia or cerebellar ataxia or motor neuron disease with hexosaminidase deficiency).

It is not the purpose of this chapter to enumerate all known biochemical defects which can cause, among other abormalities, extrapyramidal symptoms. Most of the metabolic diseases cannot be defined on clinical criteria only, but specific biochemical assays are necessary and often diagnostic. However, neuropathological examination is often either useful or necessary and confirmatory.

Disorders of Aminoacid Metabolism (Hagberg et al, 1979)

Glutaric Aciduria : defective lysine, hydroxylysine and tryptophan degradation

3-Methylglutaconic Aciduria : defective leucine degradation

Propionic Aciduria : defective valine, isoleucine, methionine, threonine, fatty acids degradation

D-Glyceric Aciduria : abnormal catabolism of serine

Homocystinuria : often cystathionine-beta-synthetase deficiency

Hyperphenylalaninemia : different enzymatic defects

Hartnup Disease : transport defect of neutral aminoacids

Neuropathological features are not specific.

Disorders of Carbohydrate Metabolism

Neuropathological features in cases of galactosemia (galactokinase or galactose-1-phosphate uridyl transferase deficiency) are not specific. Pathological examination, on the contrary, is useful to the diagnosis of glycogenoses (balloned cells with PAS-positive glycogen deposits) and is necessary to confirm the diagnosis of Lafora's disease.

Lafora Disease. Epilepsy, myoclonus and dementia are the symptoms characterizing the clinical picture of this autosomal recessive inherited disease. Inconstant other neurological symptoms include spasticity, rigidity, dysarthria and ataxia. Onset is in adolescence; death occurs within 10 years from the beginning of symptoms. EEG changes include bilaterally synchronous discharges of wave-and-spike formations.

Pathological findings are pathognomonic. Basophilic, strongly PAS-positive round intracellular inclusions are present only in neuronal perikarya, dendrites and axons. They are most frequently seen in cerebral cortex, substantia nigra, thalamus, globus pallidus and dentate nucleus. A dense core with a lighter peripheral ring is often present. Size can vary from 1 to 30 microns; the number per cell is also variable. On electron microscopy examination, a membrane is not evident. Two components are recognized: amorphous electron-dense granules and 6 nm-branched filaments (Gambetti et al, 1971). A similar material accumulate also in liver, heart, skeletal muscle, skin, which permits diagnosis in presymptomatic children (Baumann et al, 1983). The biochemical defect is still unknown. However, the storage material has been recognized as a branched polysaccharide composed of glucose (DiMauro and DeVivo, 1984).

Storage Disorders

They are transmitted as autosomal recessive trait. In many cases neuropathological examination is able to confirm the diagnosis; for some it remains the only available test. It is, however, often possible to confirm the diagnosis by specific biochemical assays.

Metachromatic leukodystrophy. Metachromatic deposits are found in urine. Peripheral nerve biopsy shows macrophages and Schwann cells containing deposits which are stained metachromatically; on electron microscopy examination, prismatic and tuffstone inclusions and zebra-like bodies are seen. Post-mortem examination of brain shows symmetrical and extensive loss of myelin in the white matter, with preservation of U-fibers. Numerous PAS-positive and metachromatically stained macrophages are present.

Sulphatide is accumulated in white matter. Assay of arylsulphatase in leucocytes, cultured fibroblasts and urine is necessary for confirmation of the diagnosis.

Globoid cell leukodystrophy (Krabbe's leukodystrophy). Peripheral nerve biopsy shows segmental demyelination; intracytoplasmic tubular profiles are seen in macrophages and rarely in Schwann cells. In the brain, marked loss of myelin with partial preservation of U-fibers is present. Astrocytic gliosis and globoid cells are seen. Globoid cells form clusters of cells in white matter, usually around blood vessels; they are strongly PAS-positive and do not show metachromasia. Enzyme assays in leucocytes and cultured fibroblasts show deficient activity of galactocerebrosidase.

GM1 gangliosidosis. Lymphocytes contain large cytoplasmic vacuoles. Skin biopsy is useful to demonstrate foamy vacuolation in sweat gland and epithelial cells, histiocytes and fibroblasts. Ballooning of neuronal cytoplasm occurs throughout the whole nervous system; the deposits are PAS-positive and metachromatically stained. Membranous cytoplasmic bodies with parallel or concentric lamellae are seen in electron microscopy. Deficiency of beta-galactosidase activity is demonstrated in serum, leucocytes and fibroblasts.

GM2 gangliosidosis. No vacuolated lymphocytes are seen. Rectal biopsy shows distended neurons of myenteric and submucosal plexuses, with membranous cytoplasmic bodies identical to those seen in GM1 gangliosidosis. Balloned neurons and glial cells, with PAS-positive and metachromatic intracytoplasmic deposits, are present throughout the central nervous system. Deficiency of hexosaminidase A or hexosaminidase A and B is demonstrated in serum, leucocytes and cultured fibroblasts.

Mucopolysaccharidosis. Microscopic and ultrastructural studies of skin and conjunctival biopsies demonstrate a storage disorder, showing the presence of pathologic material within lysosomes of cells of most tissues. PAS-positive granules, cellular vacuolation with granular or lamellar material, granulations, membranous cytoplasmic bodies identical to those of gangliosidoses, tubulovesicular inclusions are present in the different forms. However, the exact identification is not possible on morphological basis, but can be achieved by clinical and radiological examinations, enzyme assays of leucocytes or cultured fibroblasts, urinary glycosaminoglycans analysis.

Ceroid lipofuscinosis. Present classification is based on age of onset, with infantile, late-infantile, early-juvenile, juvenile and adult forms. No biochemical defect has been demonstrated. In skin biopsy, intracytoplasmic inclusions are most frequently detected in endothelial cells. They are also present in Schwann cells and neurons in peripheral nerve and rectal mucosa respectively. In infantile form, intracytoplasmic deposits are PAS-positive and show strong autofluorescence. By electron microscopy they are osmiophilic and consist of globules with a granular matrix, surrounded by a unit membrane. They can also been detected in lymphocytes. In late infantile form the storage material shows characteristic curvilinear bodies. In juvenile form "fingerprint" and curvilinear or rectilinear bodies predominate. Also in adult form curvilinear and rectilinear profiles and "fingerprint" bodies are present.

Disorders of Purine Metabolism

Lesch-Nyhan disease is an X-linked recessive disorder, due to hypoxanthine-guanine phosphoribosyltransferase deficiency in all body tissues. The rate of purine biosynthesis increases and uric acid is present in high levels in blood, urine and liquor. Severe mental retardation, spasticity and choreoathetosis develop during the first year of life. A characteristic self-mutilating behavior is present. Death results from renal failure. No distinctive pathological changes are detected in the nervous system (Hagberg et al, 1979).

Wilson Disease

Wilson disease (familial hepatolenticular degeneration) is an autosomal recessive inborn error of copper metabolism, occurring in all races. The primary defect has not yet been identified, but a failure of copper excretion through the bile is present; copper accumulates in liver, brain, kidney and cornea. The defective gene seems to be located on chromosome 13 (Frydman et al, 1983). The prevalence is 20-30 per million in Europe and United States, with a gene frequency of 0.5%.

The clinical picture, when the disease is fully established, is fairly clear. Family history of hepatic and/or neurologic dysfunctions, progressive extrapyramidal symptoms beginning during the first three decades of life, liver dysfunction, persistent aminoaciduria, cupruria, Kayser-Fleischer corneal ring are the classical features. 96% of cases show reduced or absent serum ceruloplasmin; very few cases have been reported with normal ceruloplasmin levels, suggesting the possibility of genetic heterogeneity. The neurologic manifestations are varied. Signs of basal ganglia damage often predominate, with tremor (usually "wing-beating" type), rigidity and spams. Cerebellar symptoms, convulsions, transient periods of coma, mental changes can also be associated. The sensory nervous system is spared (Walshe, 1986).

Neuropathological changes. The corpus striatum appears shrunken, with a brownish or reddish colour; cavitations are often present in the putamen. Microscopically, the putamnen shows proliferation of astrocytes; cells of Alzheimer type II (large, sometimes very large, and vesicular nuclei with one or more prominent nucleoli) are frequent; cells of Alzheimer type II (large and multinucleated) are less frequently seen. There is loss of neurons in the putamen and caudate nucleus. Lipid and iron containing cells are present around the cavitations. The globus pallidus and the subthalamic nucleus are usully relatively spared, showing reduction of neurons, Alzheimer type II cells, and Opalski cells (large cells with a finely granular or foamy cytoplasm and a small dark nucleus).

Leigh's Disease

Leigh's disease (subacute necrotizing encephalopathy) is a rare disorder usually familial, affecting infants and children; it appears to be inherited as an autosomal recessive trait. Rare adult cases have been described; they appear to be sporadic. Clinical symptoms include poor cry, impairment of feeding, arrest of psychomotor development, respiratory abnormalities. Later impairment of vision and hearing, eye mouvement abnormalities, muscular weakness and hypotonia, ataxia, dystonia and seizures can appear. Lactate and pyruvate are elevated in liquor, blood and urine. The biochemical defect(s) underlying the disease is unknown. Defective regulation of pyruvate dehydrogenase complex, deficiency of pyruvate carboxilase, and deficiency of cytochrome-c-oxidase have been reported (DeVivo, 1984).

Neuropathological findings are distinctive. Symmetrical necrosis of the grey matter with relative sparing of neurons, astrocytosis, microglial proliferation, and vascular proliferation are present in periacqueductal and periventricular areas of the brain stem. Spinal cord, cerebellum, cerebrum, basal ganglia, thalamus are often affected. Mammillary bodies are usually spared. In additon to CNS changes, cardiomyopathy, renal tubular dysfunction, growth hormone deficiency and haematopoiesis abnormalities are sometimes associated with the neurological symptoms.

MISCELLANEOUS DISORDERS

Ataxia-Telangiectasia

This is a complex familial disorder, probably transmitted as autosomal recessive trait, in which telangiectases, most prominent in the conjuntivae, are associated with cerebellar degeneration and frequent infections. Ataxia of gait beginning in infancy is the most common sign, often associated with involuntary movements of choreic or athetotic type. Other neurological abnormalities include nystagmus, dysarthria, tendon areflexia. Respiratory infections are frequent; hair and skin show premature ageing. There is a tendency to develop malignancies (especially limphomas). Immune system abnormalities, such as deficiency of IgA and IgE in the serum, delayed hypersensitivity responses and aplasia or hypoplasia of thymus are often present. Death usually intervenes before the second decade.

Pathological examination reveals that thymus is absent or rudimentary; lymphoid tissues are atrophic and gonads are hypoplasic. Dilated venules constitute the telangiectases. Atrophy of the cerebellar cortex, with loss of Purkinje and granular cells, is always present. Degeneration of the posterior columns of the spinal cord, abnormalities of posterior root ganglia and neurogenic muscolar atrophy have also been described (Sedgwick and Boder, 1972).

A defect of DNA repair mechanisms is suggested as the underlying etiologic factor (Shilosh et al, 1983).

Phakomatoses

These disorders, also called neurocutaneous dysplasias or neuro-ectodermatoses are genetic diseases involving both the skin and the nervous system. Any portion of the central and peripheral nervous system, in different combinations, may be affected by these disorders.

Tuberous sclerosis often causes, together with other symptoms and signs, myoclonic spasms, epilepsy and various extrapyramidal signs.

Neurofibromatosis, Encephalotrigeminal angiomatosis, and Incontinentia Pigmenti seldom cause extrapyramidal signs.

Hereditary Putaminal Necrosis

This is a rare familial disease, whose genetic pattern has not yet been clarified, characterized by almost isolated bilateral necrosis of the putamen and globus pallidus, or of the putamen and caudate nucleus. The onset of the first symptom varies considerably. Infantile cases seem to be most frequent; however, late-infantile, juvenile and adult onset cases have been described. The duration ranges from 3 days up to more than 30 years.

Neuropathological examination shows almost isolated necrosis, with nearly complete loss of neural elements, in the putamen and pallidus, or in the putamen and caudate nucleus, with vascular proliferation and gliosis. Substantia nigra, pons and cerebral cortex may also be affected, in various combinations, in some cases. Etiology has not yet been clarified (Druschky KF, 1986).

CHOREA ASSOCIATED WITH AUTOIMMUNE DISORDERS

Sydenham's chorea. Sydenham's chorea (acute chorea, rheumatic chorea) is a disease of childhood characterized by rapid involuntary movements, muscular weakness, hypotonia and psychological changes. Eighty per cent of cases occur in patients between the ages of 5 and 15; 75% of the patients show signs of rheumatic fever (arthritis, myocarditis, endocarditis or pericarditis) before, during or after the attack of chorea. Furthermore, serum of patients contains antibodies reacting with subthalamic and caudate nuclei in immunofluorescence assays; these antibodies also recognize membrane antigens of Group A Streptococcus (Husby et al, 1976). The course is self-limited and recovery is usually complete within 2 months. Mortality rate (due to cardiac complications) is about 2%. Recurrence is reported in 35% of cases.

Lupus-associated chorea in childhood. Chorea can be associated to systemic lupus erythematosus; in approximately 50% of these cases chorea is the presenting manifestation. The sex ratio is 6 female to one male. Twenty-five per cent of cases suffer recurrent bouts of chorea; the average duration of the attack is about 12 weeks. As the disease proceeds, convulsions, paralysis and psychosis can appear. Pathogenetic hypotheses include arteritis, small vessels degeneration and immune-complex deposition (Groothuis et al, 1977).

BASAL GANGLIA CALCIFICATIONS

Mild degree calcifications of the central nervous system, expecially of basal ganglia, are a common finding in elderly, otherwise normal, individuals; they are often seen also in arteriosclerotic vessels. They sometimes are big enough to be detected by computed tomography. Larger calcifications can be detected by plain X-rays of the skull: these cases are often symptomatic. Fifty per cent of the patients are affected by hypoparathyroidism; known causes are listed below.

BASAL GANGLIA CALCIFICATIONS (Known causes)
(Babbit et al, 1969; Troost et al, 1984)

HYPOPARATHYROIDISM:
INTOXICATIONS (Hypervitaminosis D, Lead, CO)
AFTER HEMORRAGE - AFTER INFECTION - DURING AIDS

The remainder cases have no detectable endocrine or metabolic abnormality. They are listed in the following table.

BASAL GANGLIA CALCIFICATIONS (Unknown causes)

Fahr's Disease
Idiopathic Non Familial Basal Ganglia Calcifications
Phakomatoses
Cockayne Syndrome

Fahr's disease (idiopathic familial cerebrovascular ferrocalcinosis) is characterized by severe growth disorder, mental deterioration, rigidity, tremor and blindness.
Some cases are sporadic with a wide range of clinical manifestations, according to the location and severity of brain damage: epilepsy, dementia, involuntary movements, parkinsonism and ataxia can be observed. The degree of involvement is variable; the course is slowly progressive.
Pathological examination reveals that two forms of calcification can occur: rows of small concretions along the capillary vessels and thick rings of deposit in the walls of small or medium-sized vessels. Basal ganglia and dentate nuclei of the cerebellum are the most frequent localizations.
Cockayne syndrome represents a particular form of idiopathic intracerebral calcification. Microcephaly with intracerebral calcifications is associated with growth retardation, progeria, cutaneous photosensitivity, mental retardation, pigmentary retinopathy, deafness and ataxia.
Neuropathological findings include cerebellar atrophy, brain development abormalities, demyelination in CNS and PNS; granular lysosomal inclusions have been reported in Schwann cells (Grunnet et al, 1983).

EXTRAPYRAMIDAL SYNDROMES WITHOUT PATHOLOGICAL ALTERATIONS

Dystonia Musculorum Deformans
Tics
Gilles de la Tourette Syndrome
Benign Hereditary Chorea of early onset
Diurnally Fluctuating Hereditary Progressive Dystonia

REFERENCES

Babbit DP, Tang T, Dobbs J and Berk R. Idiopathic familial cere-brovascular ferrocalcinosis (Fahr's disease) and review of differen-tial diagnosis of intracranial calcification in children. Am J Roent 105: 352-358, 1969

Baumann RJ, Kochoshis SA and Wilson D. Lafora disease: liver histopathology in presymptomatic children. Am Neurol 14: 86-89, 1983

Borit A and Herndon RM. The fine structure of plaques fibromyeli-niques in ulegyria and in status marmoratus. Acta Neuropathol 14: 304-311,1970.

Bruyn GW and Went LN. Huntington's chorea. In: Handbook of Clini cal Neurology, vol 49, Vinken PJ, Bruyn GW and Klawans HL (Eds), Elsevier, Amsterdam, 1986.

Contamin F, Escourolle R, Nick J and Mignot B. Atrophie pallido-nigro-luysienne: syndrome akinetique avec palilalie, rigidite oppo-sitionelle et catatonie. Rev Neurol 124: 107-120, 1971.

DeVivo DC. Necrotizing encephalomyelopathy and lactic acidosis. In: Merrit's Textbook of Neurology, Rowland LP (Ed), Lea & Febiger, Philadelphia, 1984.

DiMauro S and DeVivo DC. Disorders of glycogen metabolism. In: Handbook of Neurochemistry, vol 10, Lajitha A (Ed), Plenum Press, New York, 1984

Druschky KF. Hereditary putaminal necrosis (Paterson). In: Handbook of Clinical Neurology, vol 49, Vinken PJ, Bruyn GW and Klawans HL (Eds), Elsevier, Amsterdam, 1986.

Farrell DF, Clark AF, Scott CR and Wennberg RP. Absence of pyruvate decarboxylase activity in man: a cause of congenital lactic acidosis. Science 187: 1082, 1975

Frydman M, Bonne-Tamir B, Farrer LA, Conneally PM, Mogarani A, Ashbel S and Goldwich Z. Assignment of the gene for Wilson disease to chromosome 13: linkage to esterase D locus. Proc Natl Acad Sci USA 82: 1819-1821, 1985

Gambetti PL, DiMauro S, Hirt L and Blume RP. Myoclonic epilepsy with Lafora bodies. Arch Neurol 25: 483-493, 1971.

Groothuis JR, Groothuis DR, Mukhopadhyay D, Grossman BJ and Altemeier WA. Lupus-associated chorea in childhood.
Am J Dis Child 131: 1131-1134, 1977.

Grunnet ML, Zimmerman AW and Lewis RA. Ultrastructure and electro-diagnosis of peripheral neuropathy in Cockayne's syndrome.
Neurology 33:1606-1612, 1983.

Gusella JF, Wexler NS and Coneally PM. A polymorphic DNA marker genetically linked to Huntington's disease.
Nature 306: 234-238, 1983.

Hagberg B, Kyllerman M and Steen G. Dyskinesia and dystonia in neurometabolic disorders.
Neuropadiatrie 4: 305-320, 1979

Husby G, van de Rijn I, Zabriskie B, Abdin ZH and Williams RC jr. Antibodies reacting with cytoplasm of subthalamic and caudate nuclei neurons in chorea and acute rheumatic fever.
J Exp Med 144: 1094-1110, 1976

Iizuka R, Hirayama K and Maehara K. Dentato-rubro-pallido-luysian atrophy: a clinico-pathological study.
J Neurol Neurosurg Psychiat 47: 1288-1298, 1984

Jacobs JM and Le Quesne PM. Toxic disorders of the nervous system. In: Greenfield's Neuropathology, Adams JH, Corsellis JAN and Duchen LW (Eds), Edward Arnold, London, 1984.

Jellinger K. Neuroaxonal dystrophy: its natural history and re-lated disorders. In: Progress in Neuropathology, Zimmerman HM (Ed), vol 2, Grune & Stratton, New York, 1973.

Jervis GA. Huntington's Chorea in childhood.
Arch Neurol 9:244-257, 1963

Kahn J, Anderton BH, Gibb WRG, Lees AJ, Wells FR and Marsden CD. Neuronal filaments in Alzheimer's, Pick's, and Parkinson's diseases.
New Engl J Med 313: 520-521, 1985.

Konigsmark BW and Weiner LP. The olivopontocerebellar atrophies.
Medicine 49: 227-241, 1970

Larroche JC. Perinatal brain damage. In: Greenfield's Neuropatho-logy, Adams JH, Corsellis JAN and Duchen LW (Eds), Edward Arnold, London, 1984.

Lucey JF, Hibbard E, Behrman RE, Esquivel (de Gallardo) FO and Windle WF. Kernicterus in asphyxiated newborn Rhesus monkeys.
Experimental Neurology 9: 43-58, 1964.

McCormick WF and Lemmi H. Familial degeneration of the pallido-nigral system.
Neurology 15: 141-153, 1965.

Marquis P, Palmer FB, Mahoney WJ and Capute AJ. Extrapyramidal cerebral palsy: a changing view.
J Dev Behav Ped 3: 65-68, 1982

Martin WE, Loewanson RB, Resch JA and Baker AB. Parkinson's disease. Clinical analysis of 100 patients.
Neurology 23: 783-790, 1973a

Martin WE, Young WI and Anderson VE. Parkinson's disease: A genetic study.
Brain 96:495-506, 1973b

Narabayashi H, Yokochi M, Iizuka R and Nagatsu T. Juvenile parkinsonism. In: Handbook of Clinical Neurology, vol 49, Vinken PJ, Bruyn GW and Klawans HL (Eds), Elsevier, Amsterdam, 1986.

Perry TI, Norman MG, Yong VW, Whiting SH, Crichton JU, Hansen S and Kish SJ. Hallervored-Spatz disease: cysteine accumulation and cysteine dioxygenase deficiency in the globus pallidus.
Ann Neurol 18: 482-489, 1985

Sedgwick RP and Boder E. Ataxia-telangiectasia. In: Handbook of Clinical Neurology, Vinken PJ and Bruyn GW (Eds), vol 14, North-Holland, Amsterdam, 1972.

Seitelberger F. Eine unbekannte Form von infantiler Lipoid-Seicher-Krankheit des Gehirns. In: Proceeding of the First International Congress of Neuropathology, Rome, Rosenberg and Sellier, Torino, 1952

Seitelberger F. Neuroaxonal dystrophy: its relation to aging and neurological diseases. In: Handbook of clinical Neurology, vol 49, Vinken PJ, Bruyn GW and Klawans HL, (Eds), Elsevier, Amsterdam, 1986.

Shiloh Y, Tobor E and Beeker Y. Abnormal responses of ataxia-telangiectasia cells to agents that break the deoxyribose moiety of DNA via a targeted free radical mechanism.
Carcinogenesis 4:1317-1322, 1983

Stevens DL. The classification of variants of Huntington's chorea. In: Barbeau A, Chase TN and Paulson GW (Eds),Huntington's Chorea 1872-1972. Advances in Neurology, vol 1, Raven Press, New York, 1973.

Titeca J and van Bogaert L. Heredo-degenerative hemiballismus - a contribution to the question of primary atrophy of the corpus Luysii.
Brain 69:251-263, 1946.

Troost D, van Rossum A, Veiga-Pires J and Willemse J. Cerebral calcifications and cerebellar hypoplasia in two children: clinical, radiologic and neuropathological studies. A separate neurodeve-lopmental entity.
Neuropediatrics 15: 102-109, 1984

Vakili S, Drew AL, von Schuching S, Becker D and Zeman W. Hallervorden-Spatz syndrome.
Arch Neurol 34: 729-738, 1977

van Bogaert L. Etudes anatomo-cliniques des syndromes hypercineti-ques complexes. II. Un torticollis hereditaire et familial aves tremblement. Monatsschr Psychiatr Neurol 103:321-342, 1941.

van Bogaert L. Aspects cliniques et pathologiques des atrophies pallidales et pallido-luysiennes progressives.
J Neurol Neurosurg Psychiatr 9: 125-157, 1946.

Walshe JM. Wilson's disease. In: Handbook of Clinical Neurology, Vinken PJ, Bruyn GW and Klawans HL, vol 49, Elsevier, Amsterdam, 1986.

© 1987 Elsevier Science Publishers B.V. (Biomedical Division)
Extrapyramidal disorders in childhood
L. Angelini et al. editors

PROTOTYPICAL CLINICAL PICTURES AND NATURAL HISTORY OF NON PROGRESSIVE EXTRAPYRAMIDAL DISORDERS IN INFANCY AND CHILDHOOD

MASSIMO PAPINI, ANNA PASQUINELLI, NERINA LANDI, SILVIA PIACENTINI

Department of Child Neurology and Psychiatry, University of Florence, Viale GB Morgagni, 85, 50134 Florence, Italy

INTRODUCTION

Tone, Posture and Movement

Muscular tone should be considered not only in reference to the segmentary functional attitude, but also to the particular nature of the postures and movement characteristic of non progressive extra-pyramidal disorders (NPED) of childhood. Motoscopic examination (according to De Lisi, Milani–Comparetti) (1,2) consists essentially of morphological analysis of the functional significance of the postures and movements, with a special reference to the pathogenetic factors. In this way patterns (P) of posture and movement can be identified (Pattern Analysis by Milani–Comparetti) (2). This method yields results that are highly useful for identification of postural framework and the specific characteristics of motor programming pertinent to the functional structure of each different neurological forms. The contribution of Milani–Comparetti (3) to the study of non progressive forms, and that of Denny–Brown (4) to the approach to the static and progressive extrapyramidal disorders (ED), suggest that, where a posture can be recognized, tone should be considered not as a separate element but as one of the most important factors in determining the posture itself. For example, in Tetraplegic Dystonia (TeDy) the extension of the subject (S) neck when he is made to lean forward produces tonic flexion of the upper limbs. Such a complex reaction is ununderstand able if the extension and flexion tone is examined separately without considering the position of the neck. Thus tone is often the result of complex myotatic reactions, and is therefore dependent on afferent pathways determined by positions of the neck, support, etc. With motoscopic examination, it is also possible to evaluate aspects in volving modulation of postural and motor P in relation to tone, to timing and other elements, as well as to motor initiatives.

In Torsion Dystonia (ToDy), the sustained contraction of agonists and antagonists (tonic innervation by Wilson and Walshe, and by Denny-Brown) (5,6) characterizes all postural and motor functions as well as automatisms.

As regards timing, a particular posture may be assumed either extremely slowly (TeDy) or very rapidly (ToDy). Lastly, the intentional attitude, i.e. of reaching, can trigger a complex postural and motor scheme of avoiding (6) which persists as long as the intention is present.This is not a hypertonic attitude opposing with inertia and stiffness the accomplishment of a purpose, but is rather a specific behavior which involves deviation of the fovea from the image, of the hand from the object, of the foot from its support (7).

Involuntary Movements, Motor Patterns and Postures

In childhood ED, a distinction should be drawn between involuntary movements and characteristic motor P. While involuntary movements (of the choreoathetoid type, for example) are elements of interference that deviate a certain motor program from its characteristic form (as directing element: chorea; in timing: myoclonus; in strenght: ballism; etc.), motor P are characterized by a program of movement that is clearly defined in its functional attitude, with a set, unchanging morphology, alternative to normal or less pathological programs.

Some constant characteristics are present in all the main P of childhood NPED. As directing elements, we have: 1) a greater or lesser tendency to segmentary inconsistency (8), 2) rotation; as regarding timing, there are constant alterations in starting, performing, stopping, with atypical and even simultaneous reciprocal innervation such as in postural reaction modes; as regards strenght, there is that overflow of innervation (9) which confers on the movement a simultaneous appearance of effort and, for the most part, an attitude of *prestance*.

The P presenting these characteristics are generally termed "dystonic patterns", and can be recognized mainly by the movement of the upper limb and by the position assumed by the foot. The P is also characterized by the fact that it is triggered or evoked mainly by the release of complex reactions (asymmetric tonic neck reflex: ATNR) or by motor intention, depending on the clinical picture, the severity of the disorder and the phase of evolution.

The way in which the S can use the P, i.e., voluntarily trigger it in order to utilize it for movement, as occurs in TeDy, is an important characteristic dependent on the above-mentioned factors. The S can not, however, modify the P in any way, and the manner in which it is carried out depends exclusively on the nature of the disorder.

In general, motor P, more or less suitable to a particular function may be present simultaneously, and in this case there is antagonism (diadikasia = struggle to prevail according to Milani-Comparetti) (10) between the P, the most archaic of which tends to prevail. In the progressive forms evolving toward more archaic motor schemes, the most regressive scheme dominates (dominance, according to Milani-Comparetti) (11) submerging the more highly evolved P.

In a scale of severity of the disorders which can be considered as taxonomic criteria for the various childhood NPED, or in the natural history of a single progressive ED (PED), it can be observed that, as severity increases, postures become increasingly fixed and the motor schemes available decrease in number, yielding to the most archaic among them. Thus while the most specific characteristic of the lighter form is that of quality of movement, the most severe disorders are increasingly characterized by postural attitudes. "The important conclusion we wish to draw is that each type of involuntary movement is a lesser manifestation of a disorder which, when more destructive, leads to an abnormality in posture" (Denny-Brown) (6).

As regards the involuntary movements present, they have at times been confused with the motor P, from which they differ in that they are not part of the program of movement but are instead an interfering element in directional factors, in timing and in strenght. Athetosis itself is a connotational element and not a denotational one, when we consider that the characteristic aspects of an ED, a fixed one in any case, consist essentially of: 1) posture; 2) motor patterns; 3) involuntary movements. In effect the literature on double athetosis, choreoathetosis, etc., reveals extensive heterogeneity of the disorder due the fact that the postural elements of the different forms in which athetotic movements are present are determined by a wide variety of pathologies (12, 13, 6,4,14, 15) "The term athetosis applies to the movement, and not to the postural background" (Denny-Brown)(6).

PROTOTYPICAL CLINICAL PICTURES

In relation to the foregoing discussion, a clinical picture is defined as the stable result of a relationship linking, within the context of functional organization, a determined postural situation with fundamental P of movement. Involuntary movements can be present. A clinical picture is considered prototypical when there is ubiquitous consistency (in all body segments) of both postural characteristics and *repertoire* of main motor P. This consistency is not only spatial (ubiquitous) but also temporal, in the sense that other motor P are not permitted due to diadikasia. The prototypical nature of the clinical picture does not necessarily correspond to the state of current knowledge or to univocal neuropathological correlations, although TeDy, for example, is linked mainly to a putamen or corticostriatal connection damage.

In selecting prototypical clinical pictures it seems useful to apply the concepts of Denny-Brown "the general principle that in ED partial lesion leads to disturbances of movement that in greater degree become disturbances in posture" (6) in a sequence that progresses from a predominantly motor impairment to a predominantly postural one. It has been deemed useful, in considering non progressive forms, occurring moreover in childhood, to invert the order established by Denny-Brown: from the more destructured forms (mainly postural clinical aspects) to the less regressive clinical forms (mainly motorial clinical aspects).

We propose the following as prototypical clinical pictures in which the characteristics described above can be recognized:

1) apostural condition (AC); 2) II Diarchy (IIDi) of Milani-Comparetti; 3) Torsion Dystonia; 4) Tetraplegic Dystonia.

In pathological neuromotor development of NPED, there is a constant transition from one clinical picture to another. The evolutions corresponding to determined clinical pictures with phases whose modes and times are ineluctably determined, suggest that they should really be seen as step-by-step development, or a sort of "trackline journey". Moreover, a number of general extrinsic factors can prolong the stationary periods elapsing before transition to another clinical picture takes place, thus slowing down the course of progression: 1) concurrent interfering neuromotor pathologies (i.e. epilepsy); 2) mental retardation; 3) sensorial pathology or deprivation; 4) common illnesses; 5) unfavorable relational, educational and rehabilitational conditions.

The prototypical clinical pictures are rarely observed in the pure state. Within the context of NPED, in fact, mixed clinical pictures with or without involuntary movements prevail and mixed forms associated with neuromotor manifestations deriving from impairment of other systems (ataxia, etc.) are frequently present.

Apostural condition

The NPED in infancy manifest themselves in this clinical picture, which is usually included in the "floppy infant" syndrome. In some cases, this condition may persist up to the age of 4 (see conditions determining the rate of "trackline journey"). In classifying the prototypical conditions, the AC should be considered first, insofar as the pertinent organizing competence of both postural and motor P are either absent or very poor. In considering three of the main competences which the newborn should possess, i.e., 1) posture for suspension organized for its consistent balancing (16); 2) more or less complex motor patterns described by Milani-Comparetti as a *repertoire* of competence to be born (17) and 3) interactive competence well codified by Brazelton (18), the basic element indicating ED is that of postural incompetence. While the presence of hypotonia is undeniable, (physical and instrumental semeiotics), we must extrapolate from this the aspect described by

Sherrington in the following expression : the knocked-out boxer is not hypotonic but apostural. Many pathologies of the central and peripheral nervous system, both primary and secondary to a wide variety of etiologies, can result in a non-transitory "floppy infant" condition. In the pathogenesis of the AC, however, it is impairment of the postural project which is concerned rather than organizational bases (i.e., mental deficiency due to malformation of the CNS), different levels of readiness for integration (i.e., alertness), energy resources (i.e., metabolic), servo-mechanisms for achievement (i.e., II motoneuron). All of these factors, however, may tend to worsen or even disguise the postural project impairment itself.

It should be stressed that the apostural clinical picture in the strict sense, consisting of a black-out of postural competence, can evolve into conditions other than that of NPED: spastic cerebral palsy, with onset at about 3 months, and the rare Föerster syndrome (19), the so-called "atonische-astatische typus der infantilen Cerebrallähmung" where the AC becomes permanent, with signs of spasticity.

Posture. For all positions, adhesion to a plane of support determined only by body weight is observed. In passive change of position, no mechanism connecting in a functional attitude head, trunk and body segments is produced. A segment slips away and carries with it other segments (the child slips when helds).

Motor Patterns. In the purely AC we can note at the most some positions more likely to be assumed, such as the frog position and the ATNR position, at times barely discernible. Very poor, episodic, transient and incomplete labyrinthine and neck reflexes appear only at the best moments and are elicited only by repeated stimulation. Weak movements of partial flexion-extension on the support plane (wrist, ankle, knee-ankle, hip) may be present: "non functional movements" according to Milani-Comparetti (20). Over the course of time and according to the rules of the "trackline journey", sporadical motor P characteristic in form and style of the more highly developed prototypical conditions, appear. It is only later than specific postures can be elicited. This seems to demostrate that, as regards development, a motor project is more easily organized than is a postural configuration, perhaps due to the difficulty of achieving and maintaining organization in the latter condition. It follows that the factors involved in the AC in relation to the neuropathology underlying the NPED can pro bably be interpreted as maturational aspects.

Trackline Journey. The forms of "trackline journey" discussed in this paper concern only NPED in childhood, and constitute the basis for a natural history of these disorders:

1 – from 2 to 5 months, elements characteristic of the II Di appear

2 – only at the age of 12 months to 2-3 years (after the intermediate stage of the dystonic-athetosis syndrome), does ToDy become evident

3 – from 8-9 months to 2 years, characteristic elements of TeDy can be observed.

II Diarchy

Milani–Comparetti (21,20,22) has described, within the context of infantile cerebral palsies, the II Di. Some aspects attributable to this syndrome can be found in the literature on various neuromotor disorders which are difficult to classify and are for the most part of mixed types. Milani–Comparetti considers two main forms in which the supine or prone position determines a striking modification in posture. He has used the term "diarchy" to indicate the fact that dominance (from the Greek arkos=commanding) of the posture was of dual nature (from the Greek di=dual). Discussion of the I Diarchy does not fall within the scope of this paper, insofar as it involves the pyramidal system. The II Di, in our opinion, should be considered an extrapyramidal syndrome in that the postural and motor P have specific dystonic characteristics, and grimaces are present. However, Milani–Comparetti does not define the neuropathological picture and therefore no general reference to alterations of the structures and of the extrapyramidal relays is given.

The stable results of the relationship which functionally links the two predetermined postures of the II Di with the available motor P makes of it a prototypical clinical picture. The dominance of the postures as compared to the poverty of the motor P and the annihilation of any other more favorable P, place the II Di midway between the AC and the ToDy. The severe difficulty in oculomotricity, sucking, swallowing, the absence of lateral movements of the tongue, the severe dysarthria or anarthria, the impairment of the respiratory function indicate involvement of the brainstem (brainstem syndrome according to Milani-Comparetti) (22), confirming that this clinical picture should be placed at the lowest level of the functional integration after the AC.

Posture. The postural scheme is characterized by the presence of two postural P which are so strongly fixed and tyrannical as to annihilate any other more suitable choices on the antigravitational and motor level. These P cannot be evoked voluntarily, but are induced by particular positions and supports: 1) "Pseudo-Moro" pattern: (Fig.1a) elicited and maintained by placing the S lying supine on a rigid support or pushed backwards. The P consists of distressed appearance, gaping mouth, trunk leaning forward, extended trunk, crossed arms (in Jansenist crucifix position), semiflexed wrist, supinated hand, open with semiflexion of the first falanges and hyperextension of the others. Lower limbs semi-abducted, feet supinate. 2) Propulsive pattern: (Fig.1b) elicited and maintained by placing the S lying prone, suspended or vertically supported with trunk leaning forward. Pattern consists of hyperextension of the neck with possible lateral rotation, open mouth, hyperextended internally rotated elbows with flexed wrist and fisted hand, in ulnar deviation. Lower limbs extended.

Motor Patterns. Main and constantly predominating P is that of startle, with low threshold. Present, but not tyrannical nor utilizable (unlike TeDy) are the vestibular reactions, the ATNR and the Galant reflex, important for its contribution to the supporting postural asymmetry. Avoiding may be present. The reactions of support, righting, tilting, parachute are absent in the upper limbs. Therefore abrupt position change does not produce antigravity reactions, but trigger startle. The lower limbs are more available for utilization.

Functional Modes. The inability to control the head outside of the previously discussed postural schemes results in the fact that opisthotonos often asymmetric is maintained especially in the first stages, with the head falling onto the plane of support, also with the cheek resting on the arm.

Positions capable of inducing flexion of the elbow exist in the supine position, or by facilitating startle.

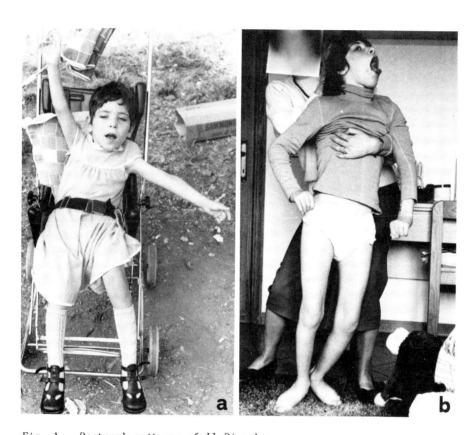

Fig. 1. Postural patterns of II Diarchy.

The sitting position may be maintained by introducing passive flexion of the knee and of the hip with acute angle, and preventing extension of the trunk with the shoulders resting against the "hopper-frame" chairback. With a table in the front and in the erect position, the arms can be kept supported, extended, adducted, internally rotated with wrists flexed, pronate with the backs of the hand resting against each other. The hands are tightly fisted if the head is hyperextended, and opening (usually of one hand only) occurs with semiflexion of the head. In this case there is lesser possibility of holding in ulnar deviation.

Standing is possible, due to the greater functionality of the lower limbs and utilization of extension synergy.

At a later stage (after the age of 10 y.), the patient, properly aided, can move around in a walker with chest rest.

Rotation may take place through abrupt unleashing of the propulsive pattern with rotation facilitated by constant asymmetry and by extension of the head.

Trackline Journey. From the AC condition there is very early transition, at the 2nd or 3rd month, to the intermediate stage in which the propulsive P appears, becoming complete by the 4th or 5th month. S with good intellective capacity, receiving physiotherapy and aided by pharmacotherapy (Trazodone inhibits startle, avoiding and favors opening of the hand and lateral movement of the tongue) (23,24,25) can utilize, albeit minimally, the diarchic P (see above) with improvement also in swallowing, phonation and breathing. The II Di presents itself not only in the non progressive forms but also in some PDE in the preterminal phase (8) confirming its position in the hierarchy of severity among the prototypical clinical pictures, according to the model of destructuration scale for ED, as described by Denny-Brown (6,4).

Torsion Dystonia.

Described by Oppenheim in 1911 (26), the non progressive ToDy is best known in the progressive form of Distonia Muscolorum Deformans, of which it represents mainly the intermediate advanced stages.

The postural/motor characteristics with the general postural P of opisthotonos and the corresponding abundance of motor P place this form midway between II Di and TeDy.

Denny-Brown (6) has described the tonic innervation in ToDy which produces a sustained and often maximum perseveration of the agonists and antagonists in posture and in movement. A slightly fluctuating dystonia (Denny-Brown) suggesting a condition of great effort, makes passive change of position almost impossible. It also produces alterations in breathing , swallowing, phonation, as well as muscular hypertrophy (i.e., of the neck), deformity (i.e., dorsoventral deformity of the foot). The intensity of the spasmus mobilis (27) may condition gradual progression of the various phases up to intense fluctuation of rigidity with the characteristic of autoexaltation, due perhaps to the effect of the afferent pathways, resulting in "bad periods" lasting for hours or months.

Posture. The general asymmetrical postural scheme, more or less evident, is that of opisthotonos in both supine and prone positions, but above all in suspension, where the flexion-extension of the neck cannot be controlled. In the supine position in addition to hyperextension of the body, the head at rest presents severe rotation, with abducted shoulders resting on the plane of support, one or both arms in the boxer position with hand clenched in fists and hypersupinated. The trunk is hyperextended and asymmetrical (projection of opisthotonos onto the plane of support), and axial inconsistency is maintained with rotation of the pelvis to the side opposite the shoulders and extension of the hips. In the prone position, the opisthotonos involves the neck and trunk, with extension of the shoulders and the hips, flexion of the elbows with external rotation of the arms, hands clenched, and sometimes flexion of the knees and inversion of the feet. On the basis of these schemes, there is a general attitude, both axial and of the limbs, toward segmentary inconsistency of the rotational type (vectorial inconsistency of rotation in the various segments gives rise to torsion).

Motor Patterns. Analysis of motor P shows the following significant aspects: 1) avoiding : differs from the classically described avoiding (6) in that the movement is not linked to the object of the vector itself, and timing is consequently altered by the number of relatively slow, repeated attempts at movement and by the sudden very fast overreaching of the target, so rapid that it can be observed only in slow-motion films (28).

The point of departure for postural asymmetry (always less evident in suspension) consists of the possibility/compulsion toward turning and keeping the neck in lateral rotation, usually extreme. Such "springy" postural recomposition may be triggered by interest taken in an object. This releases a violent reaction of avoiding involving the eyes, the head, the mouth, the trunk, and the arms, which while attempting to reach an object, are deviated away from it. The arm bends and the hand makes octopus-like or elephant-like movements (the middle finger extended, the other fingers semi-extended). The limb is pervaded by brief flexion-extension movements until the hand becomes clenched in a fist with the thumb inside (starting from a moderate pincher-grasp of semi-opposition). 2) ATNR - The lateral position of the neck brings the "jaw" arm into extension with hyperpronation and at times with internal rotation (wrist with ulnar deviation and flexion). The corresponding leg is extended, with greater latency in abduction with slight flexion of the hip. At times, the other leg crosses this one, due to abduction, flexion and internal rotation of the hip, moderate flexion of the knee and resting of the internally rotated foot on the plane of support beside the extended limb. On the other side (the "nucal" one), the shoulder is abducted with arm extended upward, elbow flexed, arm hyperpronated, wrist and fingers flexed. The position of the hand behind the neck sometimes allows the baby to play with his hair.

Spontaneous change in posture takes place through extremely rapid "springy" or chain-linked postural recomposition (spasmus mobilis). It apparently occurs as a sudden yielding of the agonistics engaged in maintaining the former muscular P, thus determining jerky movements in the opposite direction. In effect, this peculiar composing and recomposing of postures is linked to the implementation of definite postural or motor P which interfere each other in the struggle to prevail. The motor intention seems capable of triggering postural recompositions which, because of diadikasia, are often in opposition to each other and result in any case as abnormal.

Trackline Journey. ToDy is a condition appearing at about the age of 2 or 3 years after an initial aposturality and a subsequent stage characterized by dystonic postural/motor schemes.

Tetraplegic Dystonia

This condition has been described by Wilson (29) and also by Denny-Brown (6,4) , who specifies the characteristic postures and motor P . TeDy is placed at the top of the scale among these prototypical clinical pictures due to its abundance of motor P which may be capable of modifying postures and also for the fact that the motor P can be actively utilized by the S.

Rehabilitational practice has made an essential contribution to basic definition of the clinical picture which emerges by considering not so much postures as position and competence for utilization. One of the main characteristics of TeDy is that the pathology (posture and patterns) is utilized by the S to stand and move. The S has, in fact, a certain power to trigger the postural and motor schemes, although he is totally unable to modify and modulate them. This is supported by several facts: on the one hand, utilization of the ATNR for walking, albeit on the diagonal; on the other, the fact that physiotherapeutical care received by the S can also deprive him entirely of the possibility of moving, when it breaks the compensation scheme instead of utilizing it. The great effort required by the S with TeDy to stand or to carry out an act (demonstrated by his profuse sweating and by hypertrophy of the muscles of the neck), suggests that he is utilizing anti-economical mechanisms. The style of TeDy is characterized not only by the utilization of pathologic schemes, but also by the fact that those involved are mainly on the diagonal (scoliosis) (4). The S cannot aid himself in walking (which generally takes place around the age of puberty) by using his upper limbs, since it is expressly by triggering the ATNR that he is able to flex the "nucal" leg to initiate the step. Standing is achieved by finding the barycenter through hyperextension of the neck (unlike to the spastic subject), dorsal kyphosis, lumbar lordosis, extension of the hips, flexion of the knee in constant asimmetry. Another characteristic aspect is the slowness with which the S induces motor P (in contrast to the choreoathetoid condition).

Analogous to this is the variability of postures which prevents limb-deformities (apart from scoliosis, a consequences of the asymmetrical attitude).

Other general characteristics of TeDy are: moderate amimia, "sour-bitter" grimaces (especially in the presence of emotion or intention), drooling, jerky phonation (respiratory bellows impairment), tonic innervation of the eyes with difficulty in turning them from one side to the other.

Posture. Denny-Brown (4) describes dystonic posture as characterized by flexion of the upper limbs with extension of the lower limbs and extension of the trunk and the neck. "Suspension of the patient in air, with minimal body contact, accentuates the hemiplegic attitude of flexed upper limbs, extended lower, if the head is uppermost ...Inversion of the patient leads to extension of the upper limbs, flexion of the lower." (Denny-Brown) (4). In ventral suspension the upper limbs are kept extended downward, the lower limbs are flexed and the posture is accentuated by passive flexion of the neck. In dorsal suspension, the upper limbs are flexed, the lower limbs extended and the head tends to oscillate backwards. If the S lies on one side, the position assumed is the thalamic one in overall semiflection, above all in the uppermost limbs (4). For passive induction of the characteristic postures (according to Denny-Brown) (4), these S must remain for a long time in the position which induces the posture, due to the slowness of their reactions. The postures are moreover very sensitive to suspension and are also conditioned by support, i.e., by the body contact with the plane on which it rests. In addiction, the posture is often constantly asymmetrical due to the predominance of the ATNR.

Motor Patterns. The motor P present (4) and predominating in TeDy are: 1) mainly ATNR , as scheme conditioning and determining postural/motor states; in addition , 2) vestibular reactions (observable with postures in suspension), 3) avoiding (6,28,30), 4) grasping (tonic grasp reflex), 5) Galant reflex.

Trackline Journey. An early characteristic is the supine attitude of the feet in the downward parachute without "scissoring", or similarly, the persistence and dominance of the ATNR. Also characteristic is the tendency to fall backward. These signs emerge at about the age of 8 months, after a long phase of aposturality, and tend to assume the typical characteristics at about the age of 2 years.

DISCUSSION

In classifying prototypical clinical pictures according to severity, from the most severe condition to the least severe one, these aspects are to be pointed out:

A) when postural tyranny establishes itself, the possibility of eliciting motor P vanishes;

B) two significant characteristics of the motor P may be observed: 1- the possibility that a motor P may enter into dynamic equilibrium with a postural one and, therefore, the functional-adaptational utility of balancing between the two; 2- the possibility that a P may be utilized by the S (Tab.1)

TABLE 1

Graduation of severity of clinical pictures: examples of balancing between motor and postural P and utilization of a motor pattern.

Clinical picture:	AC >	II Di >	ToDy >	TeDy
Balancing of the extension pattern by:	–	Galant r.	ATNR	Flexion synergy P
Utilization and influence of ATNR:	negligible	without influence	tyrannic	utilized

The definition of these four prototypical clinical pictures, based on pattern analysis of posture and movement P, has been proposed for the purpose of providing points of orientation within the context of the mixed clinical pictures and of the mixed forms, which constitute the great majority of PED and NPED. The term <u>mixed clinical picture</u> of NPED regards both the mono or bilateral concurrent presence of one or the other clinical picture as well as concomitant involuntary movements (i.e. athetosis). In <u>mixed forms</u> instead there may exist (mono or bilaterally) manifestations of impairment of a wide variety of neuromotor systems. It has been found useful, also in the mixed forms, to apply the concepts of tyranny and diadikasia in order to understand dynamic equilibrium in relation to balancing of modules, patterns and postures belonging to different pathologies. The modules (i.e. ataxia) or the motor P (i.e. spasticity) characteristic of the various pathologies can be submerged by the postural tyranny of the more severe clinical pictures.

The rating scales of ED for evaluation of therapeutic effects are, in our opinion, useful mainly for verifying the quantity of involuntary movements and the timing of the movement (akinesia, on-off, etc.). Pattern analysis introduces the possibility of evaluating the qualitative element, i.e. the availability of one of the motor P in the *repertoire* at the disposal of the S. It is expressly the remission or the diminution of a P which may be at the basis of a qualitative improvement, as in the case of reduction of avoiding (28,30) and of startle (25). Lastly, pattern analysis is useful for early identification of postural and motor P which allow us to recognize a clinical picture that is evolving from the AC, by precocious delineation of important diagnostic-prognostic aspects. In PED, moreover, pattern analysis offers important references for verifying deviations from the predicted prognosis (11,20), for indicating the course of evolution and for offering suggestions as to relief therapy.

ACKNOWLEDGEMENTS

This work is dedicated to the memory of Professor Adriano Milani-Comparetti, from whom derive the main concepts and contributions. We wish to thank Doctors ML Fantini and EA Gidoni for their constant, invaluable collaboration.

This work was supported by Grant CNR No 86.01891.56.

REFERENCES

1. De Lisi L (1931) Arch gen Neurol Psichiat Psicoanal 12:271

2. Milani-Comparetti A, Gidoni EA (1967) Develop Med Child Neurol 9: 625-628

3. Milani-Comparetti A (1965) Infanzia anormale 64:597-628

4. Denny- Brown D (1968) In: Vinken PJ, Bruyn GW (eds) Handbook of Clinical Neurology. North-Holland, Amsterdam, 6:133-172

5. Wilson SAK, Walshe FMR (1914) Brain 37:199-246

6. Denny-Brown D (1962) The Basal Ganglia and Their Relation to Disorders of Movement. Oxford University Press, London

7. Papini M, Pasquinelli A, Landi N (1987) In: Proceed 1a Riunione Gruppo di Studio sui "Disordini del Movimento" Soc It Neurol,CNR, Roma, 3-4 Aprile 1987, p 45

8. Papini M, Martinetti MG, Pasquinelli A (1982) G Neuropsich Età Evol II, 4:349-357

9. Föerster O (1921) Z Neurol Psychiat 73:1-169

10. Milani- Comparetti A (1981) Riv Neurobiol 28:572-577

11. Milani- Comparetti A, Gidoni EA (1971) Neuropsichiatria Infantile 121:252-271

12. Carpenter MB (1950) Arch Neurol Psychiat 63:875-901

13. Twitchell TE (1959) J Nerv Ment Dis 129:105-132

14. Foley J (1983) J Neurol Neurosurg Psychiat 46:289-298

15. Salam-Adams M, Adams RD (1986) In: Vinken PJ, Bruyn GW (eds) Handbook of Clinical Neurology. North-Holland, Amsterdam, 49:381-389

16. Peiper A (1963) Cerebral Function in Infancy and Childhood. Consultants Bureau, New York

17. Milani-Comparetti A (1981) Seminars of Perinatology 5:183-189

18. Brazelton TB (1973) Neonatal Behavioral Assessment Scale. Heineman Medical Books, London

19. Föerster O (1909) Dtsch Arch Klin Med 98:216

20. Milani-Comparetti A (1982) Prospettive in Pediatria 48:305-314

21. Milani-Comparetti A (1978) Méd Hyg 36:2024-2029

22. Milani-Comparetti A (1983) In: Agnoli A, Bertolani G (eds) Proceed 10a Riunione Lega It contro M di Parkinson e M Extrapiramidali, Pavia, Ottobre 1983."D Guanella" Publ,Roma, pp 290-295

23. Papini M, Milani-Comparetti A, Gidoni EA, Martinetti MG, Pasquinelli A, Fantini ML (1981) In: De Negri M (ed) Comptes rendus du 2ème Congrès de la Société de Neurologie Infantile, Genova, 4-6 Déc 1981. Gaslini, Genova, 13:189

24. Papini M, Martinetti MG, Pasquinelli A (1982) It J Neurol Sci 2:161-162

25. Papini M, Milani-Comparetti A, Gidoni EA, Martinetti MG, Pasquinelli A (1981) Riv Neurobiol 27:591-596

26. Oppenheim (1911) Neurol Zentralbl 30:1090-1107

27. Gowers WR (1876) Med Chir Trans 59:271-320

28. Papini M, Pasquinelli A, Costa P, Armellini M, Piacentini S, Chelazzi C, Frosini R (1984) In: Neetens A (ed) Proceed Neuro-Ophthalmology Joint World Meeting INOS V and WFN VII, Antwerp/Belgium, May 14-18 1984. University of Antwerp U.I.A., Antwerp, pp 139-143

29. Wilson SAK (1912) Brain 34: 295-509

30. Papini M, Pasquinelli A, Costa P, Landi N (1986) In: Calamoneri F, Mangano S, Sciortino F (eds) Proceed XII Cong Naz Soc It Neuropsichiatria Infantile, Cefalù, 1-4 Ottobre 1986. Ediprint, Siracusa, p. 351

© 1987 Elsevier Science Publishers B.V. (Biomedical Division)
Extrapyramidal disorders in childhood
L. Angelini et al. editors

GENETIC METABOLIC DISEASES WITH EXTRAPYRAMIDAL SIGNS AND SYMPTOMS

STEFANO DI DONATO°, GRAZIELLA UZIEL°°

°Divisione di Biochimica e Genetica del Sistema Nervoso, °°Divisione di Neuropsichiatria Infantile, Istituto Neurologico "C. Besta, via Celoria 11, 20133 Milano, (Italy)

INTRODUCTION

Extrapyramidal signs and symptoms are most strikingly seen in degenerative disorders of the Basal Ganglia of still unknown etiology and pathogenesis. Dystonia, dyskinesia, including parkinsonism and choreoathetosis, and myoclonus are seen in different association, in the Progressive Childhood Dystonias, Choreas and Athetosis. These disorders include juvenile Huntington disease, Wilson disease, dystonia musculorum deformans, juvenile Parkinson disease, Familial Calcification of the Basal Ganglia. Moreover, some genetic metabolic disorders of known etiology, may present as Dystonic-Diskinetic syndromes (DDS) and therefore enter in the diffential diagnosis of the Progressive Childhood Dystonias (1). Metabolic disorders characterized by progressive DDS include specific defects in aminoacid, carbohydrate and purine metabolism, some of the lipid storage diseases due to lysosomal pathology, and some defects of mitochondrial enzymes (2).

In a few of these metabolic disorders of known origin, DDS is the major clinical sign, while in most metabolic diseases DDS may appear in the clinical picture associated to other symptoms, which clearly orient the diagnosis. This review deals essentially with metabolic disorders in which the main clinical presentation is progressive DDS in infancy and childhood.

Metabolic diseases with DDS

Genetic metabolic diseases affect different metabolic pathways in the brain and cause neuronal death or neuronal disfunction in definite areas of the Basal Ganglia by poorly understood mechanisms. These may include :

a) disturbances of the brain content of metals, as in Wilson disease

b) disturbances of osmotic and acid-base homeostasis, as in the organic acidurias

c) modification of synthesis, uptake and catabolism of critic neurotransmitters, as in disorders of phenylalanine, tyrosine and tryptophan metabolism

d) distorsions of the neuronal geometry, as in the lipid storage disease.

In some instances different events cooperate in disturbing the structure and the function of the Basal Ganglia, as in the case of mitochondrial disorders, in which both intracellular alterations in the redox state of the flavin and nicotinamide coenzymes and altered tissue and vascular responses to hypoxia, may contribute to neuronal pathology (3).

Table 1 shows the genetic metabolic diseases clinically characterized by progressive DDS. Table 2 shows the metabolic diseases in which DDS may be present but is not pathognomonic of the disease.

TABLE 1

GENETIC METABOLIC DISEASES WITH OVERT DYSTONIC - DYSKINETIC SYNDROME

1 . Aminoacid metabolism

    a - glutaric aciduria type I
    b - hyperphenylalaninemias

2 . Purine metabolism

    a - HPRT deficiency (Lesch-Nyhan syndrome)

3 . Lysosomal diseases

    a - juvenile dystonic lipidosis
    b - GM_1 gangliosidosis (dystonic phenotype)
    c - GM_2 gangliosidosis (dystonic phenotype)
    d - α neuraminidase deficiency (CRS-myoclonus syndrome)

4 . Mitochondrial diseases

    a - pyruvate dehydrogenase deficiency
    b - cytochrome-c-oxidase deficiency

TABLE 2

GENETIC METABOLIC DISEASES WITH OCCASIONAL DYSTONIC - DYSKINETIC
SYNDROME

1 . Aminoacid metabolism

    a - maple syrup urine disease
    b - isovaleric acidemia
    c - 3methyl crotonylCoA carboxylase deficiency
    d - 3methyl glutaconylCoA hydratase deficiency
    e - 3 HMG-CoA lyase deficiency
    f - acetoacetylCoA lyase deficiency
    g - propionic acidemia
    h - multiple carboxylase deficiency
    i - phenylketonuria
    l - cystinuria
    m - homocystinuria

2 . Lysosomal diseases

    a - Krabbe disease
    b - metachromatic leukodystrophy
    c - Gaucher disease
    d - fucosidosis
    e - Salla disease
    f - mucopolysaccaridosis III
    g - mucolipidosis I

3 . Miscellaneous metabolic disorder

    a - pyruvate - carboxylase deficiency
    b - galattosemia
    c - respiratory chain defects

The known biochemical and genetic heterogeneity of the metabolic disorders makes this
distinction somewhat artificial : it is therefore intended that the phenotypic expression
varies in different families due to both genetic and epigenetic factors.

1 . Amino acid metabolism

a) Glutaric aciduria type I (GA I)

  GA I is a disease of infancy characterized by recurrent episodes of metabolic acidosis
and progressive neurological deterioration with choreathetosis and dystonia, mental
retardation and spastic quadriparesis (1). The disease is inherited in an autosomal
recessive fashion. The primary metabolic defect in GA I is thougtht to be a deficiency of
the mitochondrial glutarylCoA dehydrogenase : the activity of this enzyme is in fact

68

markedly low in the patient's liver, leukocytes and cultured fibroblasts (5, 6). The progressive movement disorder seen in GA I patients is associated to striatal necrosis : pathological studies show a severe symmetrical distruction of the putamen and lateral margins of the caudate (1), associated with fatty changes in liver, kidney and myocardium.

The marked metabolic acidosis seen in these subjects is due to large accumulation in body fluids of glutaric, glutaconic and 3-OH glutaric acids (4, 6) : the presence of these two latters metabolites is not immediately understood. Indeed, low activity of glutarylCoA dehydrogenase would simply lead to the accumumulation of glutaric acid, an intermediate in the catabolism of tryptophan, lysine and hydroxylysine. It is believed that the flavoprotein is able to catalyze the conversion of glutarylCoA to crotonylCoA by two successive reactions, namely dehydrogenation of glutarylCoA to glutaconylCoA and decarboxylation of glutarylCoA (7), as shown in figure 1.

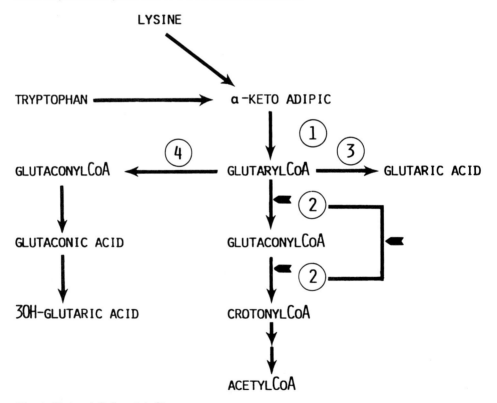

Fig. 1 Glutaryl CoA metabolism
1 = α-ketoacid dehydrogenase; 2 = glutarylCoA dehydrogenase (mitochondrial); 3 = glutaryl CoA thyolase; 4 = glutaryl CoA oxidase (peroxisomal); ◀ = site of the metabolic block in GA I

This figure hypothizes alternative routes for the metabolism of glutarylCoA in case of glutarylCoA dehydrogenase deficiency : it is seen that glutaconic and 3-OH glutaric acids found in patients' urine could origin by peroxisomal oxidation of glutarylCoA, as recently reported (8).

The neurodegenerative picture in GA I has not been elucidated, but it has been suggested that glutarate can be specifically toxic to Basal Ganglia. Indeed glutarate and glutamate are chemical analogs, and glutarate might be able to impair glutamate decarboxylation to GABA, by acting as a competitive inhibitor of glutamate decarboxylase, or interfere with selective glutamate uptake by specific receptors (1, 6). There is no treatment of the disease except dietary treatment, low in lysine and tryptophan : however, some patients with GA I, may develop secondary carnitine deficiency, as do patients with other organic acidurias (9), and oral carnitine supplementation may be helpful (10).

b) Hyperphenylalaninemias

Phenylketonuria (PKU) is a classic example of genetic metabolic disorder : it is characterized by autosomal recessive inheritance, increased levels of phenylalanine in body fluids, and deficiency of the enzyme phenylanine hydroxylase, leading to mental retardation that can be prevented by the appropriate dietary restriction of phenylalanine (11).

Hyperphenylalaninemias with defects in the phenylalanine hydroxylase system, other than phenylalanine hydroxylase itself, i.e. deficiency of dihydropteridine reductase (DHPR), the enzyme able to catalyze the conversion of dihydropteridine to the active tetrahydrobiopterine (B_4), or to the biopterine synthesis have been reported (12).

These forms of hyperphenylalaninemia were identified since the patients were unresponsive to dietary restriction of phenylalanine, and deteriorated neurologically with progressive myoclonus, dystonia, spasticity and seizures. Since the levels of phenylalanine were controlled in these patients, it was suggested that the DDS might be the results of alterated biosynthesis of critical neurotransmitters. Figure 2 shows the role of B_4 in phenylalanine, tyrosine and tryptophan metabolism and indicates that impairements in B_4 availability can interfere with the synthesis of serotonine, noradrenaline and dopamine, since B_4 is the coenzyme of the hydroxylases active in catecolamine biosynthesis. In agreement with this hypothesis, patients with hyperphenylalaninemias due to DHPR deficiency or defective biopterine synthesis, excrete very low amounts of 5 hydroxyindolacetic (5HIAA), homovanillyc (HVA) and vanillymandelic (VMA) acids, the metabolites of the mentioned catecolamines (13). Moreover, these patients respond clinically to DOPA, carbidopa and 5 OH tryptophan supplementation better than to phenylalanine restriction (12, 13, 14).

B_4 BIOSYNTHESIS

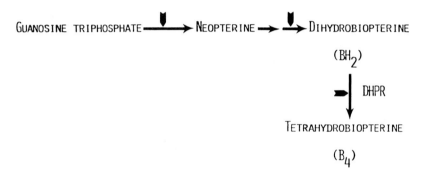

CATECOLAMINES BIOSYNTHESIS

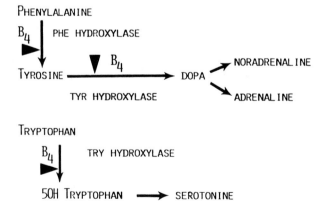

Fig. 2 Hyperphenylalaninemias
DHPR = dihydropteridine reductase; ➡ defects of B_4 biosynthesis; ▶ = defects of catecolamines metabolism due to altered B_4 biosynthesis (from ref. 13, modified)

The biochemical diagnosis of the hyperphenylalaninemias is complex due to the extensive clinical and biochemical heterogeneity.

Several criteria help in the diagnosis of the three major biochemical phenotypes, i.e. deficiency of phenylalanine hydroxylase, deficiency of DHPR and deficiency of biopterim synthesis. These two latters disorders show increased levels of blood phenylalanine and low urinary 5HIAA, HVA and VMA; moreover, the activity of phenylalanine hydroxylase is normal in the patients' cells (13, 14). The normal or low activity of DHPR can discriminate the two forms with altered B_4 metabolism (14).

Regional studies of the brain have shown that B_4 is concentrated in the striatum and other sites of monoamine synthesis suggesting that B_4 concentration in specific areas may be rate-limiting for the synthesis of serotonine and dopamine (15).

Recently acute intravenous administration of B_4 in patients with primary dystonias was shown to be able to improve some of the clinical symptoms and signs in about 50% of the subjects treated, suggesting a role for this cofactor in'the pathogenesis of primary dystonias and in their possible treatment (15).

2 . Purine metabolism

a) Lesch Nyhan syndrome

The Lesch-Nyhan syndrome (LNS) is an X-linked disease characterized by compulsive self-mutilation, developmental retardation, spasticity and choreoathetosis (16). There is an overproduction of uric acid due to an accelerated rate of de novo purine biosynthesis : this is secondary to a deficiency of the enzyme hypoxantine-guanine phosphoribosyltransferase (HPRT), for which human genetic studies indicate that the structural gene is located on the X chromosome (17). HPRT is a purine salvage enzyme which converts preformed purine bases, hypoxantine and guanine, to their respective nucleotides : indeed it provides an alternate pathway to de novo synthesis of inosine and guanosine monophosphates (IMP and GMP) by catalizing the transfer of phosphoribose from 5-phosphoribosyl-1-pyrophosphate to hypoxantine or guanine bases to yield IMP or GMP (18).

At difference with the patients with mitocondrial encephalomyopathies (MEs) due to cytocrome-c-oxidase deficiency (see below), neuropatological studies in brains from patients with LNS demonstrate no appreciable morphological abnormality of the brain, including the Basal Ganglia (16) : however in these patients DDS is one of the pathognomonic neurological signs, while it is rarely observed in MEs, as later discussed. It has been suggested that discrete biochemical alterations rather than substantial pathological changes underlie CNS sufference in LNS (16, 19).

A detailed biochemical study of brain neurotransmitters and HPRT activity was performed by Lloyd and coworkers (16) in order to ascertain this hypothesis. The authors found that the level of HPRT activity in the brain from three patients was lower than 1 per cent of control and that all aspects of the function of dopamine-neuron terminals in the striatum were decreased to 10 to 30 per cent of the control values. Striatal glutamate decarboxylase activity and serotonine levels were normal, or increased, while striatal choline acetyltransferase activity was low. The authors concluded that the neurological symptoms observed in LNS, namely choreoathetosis, was due to the dysruption of the balance between the functions of GABA, dopamine and acetylcholine neurons in the extrapyramydal system (16).

An intriguing observation, in respect to this hypothesis, is that the Basal Ganglia have the highest HPRT activity and the lowest phosphoribosyl pyrophosphatase (PRPP) activity (PRPP is the first enzyme in de novo pathway of purine biosynthesis). These findings indeed suggest that the Basal Ganglia may be very dependent on HPRT for the maintenance of a constant level of intracellular purine biosynthesis (19).

3 . Lysosomal diseases

a) Juvenile dystonic lipidosis

An unusual form of neurovisceral storage disease was described in detail by Karpati and coworkers in 1977 in two unrelated boys of 11 and 13 years of age (20). Both patients had normal development, but later showed a neurological disorder characterized by dystonia and involuntary movements with facial grimacing, dysarthria and splenomegaly : epilepsy, visual impairment and dementia were absent (20). Pathological studies revealed a marked lipid storage in splenic histocytes and visceral neurons : the neuronal inclusions were different from the splenic inclusions since they resembled the membranous cytosplenic bodies (MCB) seen in Tay Sach's disease or the zebra bodies seen in the mucopolysaccharidoses. The disease resembled pathologically the juvenile type of Niemann Pick disease, but the activity of sphyngomyelinase in leukocyte was normal (20). These patients resembled a few others patients previously reported in the literature (21, 22). A precise biochemical diagnosis was not reached in any of these patients; even the demonstration of specific pathological involvement of the Basal Ganglia is lacking since autopsies were not performed (20).

b) GM_1 gangliosidosis

Typical GM_1 gangliosidosis is a pediatric disorder with neurovisceral storage, rapid neurological deterioration and death in the early infancy. Juvenile and adult forms of GM_1 gangliosidosis show different phenotypes with ataxia, seizures, multiple dysostosis and cherry-red spot at the macula variably associated in relation to the extensive biochemical heterogeneity of the disease (23).

Adult GM_1 gangliosidosis, however, can be specifically characterized by a dystonic phenotype (24, 25). This disease begins generally in childhood with slowly progressive dystonia and mild intellettual deterioration : myoclonus seizure and macular cherry-red spot are absent. The dystonic syndrome becomes progressively incapacitating with torticollis, facial grimacing, explosive speach and oculogyric crisis. β-galactosidase activity is very low in patients' tissues and leukocytes (24). The major and significative differences between these adult patients with DDS and the infantile and late GM_1 gangliosidosis are the pathological changes : in the former they are localized in the Basal Ganglia with relative sparing of the cerebral cortex, thus providing a correlation with DDS (24). Some degree of clinical heterogeneity is present in adult GM_1 gangliosidosis, as exemplified by a Japanese family in which, of three affected members, one had a progressive incapaciting DDS, while other two affected brothers had only occasional dystonia (26).

c) GM_2 gangliosidosis

GM_2 gangliosidosis is the best known neuronal lipidosis. This autosomal recessive disorder can be due to at least two different biochemical phenotypes : a) Tay Sach's disease, due to deficiency of the β-hexosaminidase A isoenzyme; the mutation is on chromosome 15 at the α-locus, the gene locus coding for the α-subunit of the enzyme;

b) Sanhdoff disease, due to the deficiency of the β-hexosaminidase A and B isoenzymes; the mutation is at the locus on chromosome 5, the gene locus coding for the β-subunit of the enzyme, which is common to both A and B isoenzymes (27,28).

The spectrum of phenotypes resulting from storage of GM_2 ganglioside, the main substrate of ß-hexosaminidase, is quite large. It includes the classical infantile forms with seizures, dementia and cherry-red spots at the macula the late infantile and juvanile forms with dementia, ataxia, seizures and myoclonus and the late-onset forms with spinocerebellar degeneration, motor neuron disease or amyotrophic lateral sclerosis-like phenotypes (27). Juvenile and adult forms of β-hexosaminidase deficiency with complex neurological symptoms including dystonia have been rarely reported (29, 30). Meek and coworker (31) however, reported on a juvenile form of GM_2 gangliosidosis specifically characterized by progressive dystonia. The age of onset was 2 1/2 years and the clinical picture was dominated, in this 10-years-old boy, by dystonic and choreiform movements, suggesting Basal Ganglia involvement : progressive dementia was associated to the DDS (29). Serum, leukocyte and fibroblast activities of β-hexosaminidase A were markedly reduced in the patient, thus confirming that this particular phenotype was due to mutation at the α-locus (31). A similar patient, a 10 year old girl, with progressive psycomotor disfunction and dystonic posturing had low activity of both β-hexosaminidases A and B, suggesting a mutation at the β-locus (32).

d) Cherry-red spot myoclonus syndrome

A slowly progressive neurological syndrome that combines action sensitive and stimulus sensitive myoclonus, cherry-red spot at the macula and no evidence of early dementia has been described as a distinct clinical entity by Rapin and coworkers (33). J. O'Brien proved that the biochemical defect in this rare lysosomal disorder was a deficiency of lysosomal α-neuraminidase, an enzyme able to hydrolyze sialic acid from both glycoprotein and glycolipid substrates (34). Some of the patients subsequently described positively responded to serotonine precursor supplementation : one of our patients was treated along 18 months with high doses of oral 5-hydroxytriptophan with prolonged benefical effects on myoclonus (35).

4 . Mitochondrial diseases

The mitochondrial encephalomyopathies (ME) are a ill-defined group of diseases in which there is evidence of : a) muscle weakness; b) variable central nervous system involvement; c) morphological and/or biochemical mitochondrial abnormalities (36). In rare instances patients with MEs have DDS, associated to pathological and biochemical evidence of Basal Ganglia involvement; sometime there is an association of DDS with a deficiency of a mitochondrial enzyme; sometime the pathological involvement of the Basal Ganglia is associated to mitochondrial dysfunction. Biochemically, the MEs are considered to fall into two main groups : a) defects of substrate utilization; b) defects of the respiratory chain. Among the first group we will consider the pyruvate dehydrogenase complex (PDHC) deficiencies and among the second group the citochrome-c-oxidase (COX) deficiencies : both are characterized by extensive phenotypic variation.

a) PDHC deficiencies

The PDHC catalyzes the irreversible oxidation of pyruvate to acetylCoA, which is either oxidized in the tricarboxylic acid cycle or used for biosynthetic purposes. The enzyme complex is composed in mammalian tissues of three catalytic and two regulatory components. The catalytic enzymes are pyruvate decarboxylase , $PDH-E_1$, dihydrolipoyl transacetylase, $PDH-E_2$, and dihydrolipoyl dehydrogenase, $PDH-E_3$; the regulatory enzymes are PDH kinase, which catalyzes the Mg-ATP-dependent phosphorylation of E_1 with subsequent inactivation of PDHC, and PDH-phosphatase which is responsible for dephosphorylation and activation of the complex (figure 3) (38). Over 50 patients with lactic acidosis and deficiency of PDHC have been reported in the literature with a wide variety of clinical symptoms such as Friedreich's ataxia, intermittent ataxia, acute infantile lethal acidosis, mitochondrial myopathy and Leigh's syndrome. Some of the phenotypes reported were characterized by DDS.

Blass et al firstly described in 1970 a 8 years old boy with "intermittent movement disorder", characterized by attacks of cerebellar dysfunction, choreoathetosis and dystonic posturing, and slight elevation of blood pyruvate, lactate and alanine. Pyruvate decarboxylase activity was low in patient's leukocytes and fibroblasts (39).

A retarded boy of 8.5 years of age, with dystonic posturing and continous choreoathetoid movements was later described by the same authors (40). This patient had a deficiency of PDHC in fibroblast, localized at the level of the second catalytic component, PDH, E_2 (40).

Pride and coworkers, conversely, described a 18 months girl with progressive psychomotor retardation, myoclonus, seizures and spasticity with PDHC low in the brain, but normal in fibroblast, leukocyte and liver (41).

Leigh's syndrome

Leigh's subacute necrotizing encephalomyelopathy (SNE) is a clinically and biochemically heterogeneous disorder of infancy and early childhood, characterized neuropathologically by necrotizing lesions of the deep midline structures. Extrapyramidal signs are sometime present in patients of older age 42), but they are not frequent in most of the patients in spite of the fact that brain pathology shows pathognomonic lesions of the Basal Ganglia, at the internal part of the thalamus and caudate nucleus (43). The neuropathological findings have a clear counterpart in vivo, and CT scan of the brain reveals typical bilateral simmetrical lesions of the medial talamus and the putamen (44).

After the first report of Farmer and coworkers in 1973 (45), pyruvate decarboxylase deficiency in Leigh's syndrome has been reported by some authors (46, 47). We have seen five patients with PDH deficiency : some of these patients did show clinical involvement of the Basal Ganglia (table 3).

TABLE 3

PATIENTS WITH PDHC DEFICIENCY IN CULTURED FIBROBLASTS

Subjects	Blood[••] lactate	Clinical DDS	PDHC[•] non activated	activated
F.D.	3.1	±	0.07	0.18
DA.G[•]	3.9	++	0.52	0.76
D.E.[•••]	4.2	++	0.30	0.28
S.S.[•••]	2.5	±	0.45	0.46
V.V.[•••]	3.1	±	0.90	0.84
Controls (12)	< 2.0	–	2.11 ± 1.2	4.0 ± 2.3

[•]PDHC activity is given as nanomoles pyruvate oxidized/min/mg fibroblast protein
[••]Blood lactate is given in mmoles/l
[•••]Patients with low PDHC activity and impaired PDHC activation

The correlations between PDHC deficiency and Basal Ganglia dysfunction have not been investigated and are therefore unknown. It can be speculated, however, that PDHC deficiency may go along with low synthesis of acetylcholine (48) in subsets of neurons with an imbalance between the levels of acetylcholine and GABA and catecolamine in the striatum. The relationships between PDHC activity and acetylcholine synthesis are shown in figure 3.

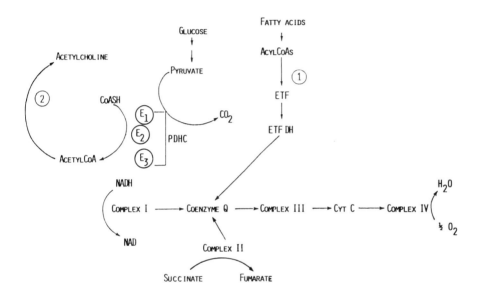

Fig. 3 Glucose and fatty acid oxidation and the respiratory chain
1 = primary acylCoA dehydrogenases; 2 = choline acetyltransferase; E_1, E_2, E_3 = catalytic components of the pyruvate dehydrogenase complex (see text)

It is noteworthy to remember that Leigh's syndrome has been associated to defects different from PDHC deficiency, such as pyruvate carboxylase and cytochrome-c-oxidase deficiencies (see below).

b) Cytochrome-c-oxidase deficiency

Cytochrome-c-oxidase (COX) is the last enzyme complex (complex IV) of the respiratory chain and its fundamental function is that of transferring electron equivalents from reduced cytochrome-c to molecular oxigen. COX function and that of other components of the respiratory chain and of related mitochondrial enzymes, including PDHC, are shown in figure 3.

Leigh's syndrome

COX deficiency, similarly to PDHC deficiency, is expressed in humans with different clinical and biochemical phenotypes (49). Fatal infantile mitochondrial myopathy with renal insufficiency and lactic acidosis, floppy infant's syndrome with lactic acidosis and cardiomyopathy, benign mitochondrial myopathy with reversible muscle cytochrome-c-oxidase deficiency have been described (50). More recently, five unrelated patients with neuropathologically proven Leigh's SNE have been reported (51). All these patients had COX deficiency in multyple tissues, namely the brain, muscle and kidney. The COX activity in the brain ranged between 15 and 32% the normal mean, while the activities of other mitochondrial enzymes, including PDHC, and other subcomplexes of the respiratory chain were in the normal range (51).

COX is a complex enzyme composed of 13 subunits, of which 3 (subunits I to III) are encoded to by mitochondrial DNA, while the other 10 are encoded to by nuclear DNA (52). Since Leigh's syndrome is an autosomal recessive disease, it is suggested that defects of nuclear encoded subunits underlie COX deficiency in these patients.

Interestingly, there is another mitochondrial disease associated to low COX activity and characterized by myoclonus, epilepsy, ataxia, weakness and mental deterioration, the Myoclonus-Epilepsy with Ragged-Red fibers (MERRF) (53). This disease is transmitted in a non-mendelian maternal inheritance : low activity of COX was found and a defect in a mitochondrially encoded subunit of complex IV has been suggested (54).

ACKNOWLEDGEMENTS

This work has been supported by the grant CT 86.02020.56 of the Consiglio Nazionale delle Ricerche (CNR), Roma, Italy.

REFERENCES

1. Leibel RL, Shih VE, Goodman SI et al (1980) Neurology 30: 1163-1168

2. Hagberg B, Kyllerman M, Steen G (1979) Neuropaediatrie 10: 305-320

3. Di Donato S (1985) In : Berra B, Mollica F, Pavone L, Rapelli S : Progress in Mitochondrial, Mendelian and Chromosomal Disorders. Persp Inher Met Dis 6, pp 39-51

4. Goodman SI, Markey SP, Moe PG et al (1975) Biochem Med 12: 12-21

5. Goodman SI, Kohlhoff JG (1975) Biochem Med 13: 138-140

6. Gregersen N, Brandt NJ, Christensen F et al (1977) J Pediat 90: 740-745

7. Hyman DB, Tanaka K (1984) J Clin Invest 73: 778-784

8. Vamecq J, de Hoffmann F, Van Hoof F (1985) Eur J Bioch 146: 663-669

9. Di Donato S, Rimoldi M, Garavaglia B, Uziel G (1984) Clin Chim Acta 139: 13-21

10. Seccombe DW, James L, Booth F (1986) Neurology 36: 264-267

11. Scriver CR, Clow CL (1980) N Engl J Med 303: 1336-1342

12. Smith J, Clayton BE, Wolff OH (1975) Lancet 1: 1108-1111

13. Berlow S (1980) Pediatrics 65: 837-839

14. Kaufman S (1980) Pediatric 65: 840-841

15. Le Witt PA, Miller LP, Levine RA et al (1986) Neurology 36: 760-764

16. Lloyd KG, Hornykiewicz O, Davidson L (1981) N Engl J Med 305: 1106-1111

17. Caskey CT, Kruh GD (1979) Cell 16: 1-9

18. Seegmiller JE, Rosenbloom FM, Kelley WN (1967) Science 155: 1682-1685

19. Howard WJ, Kerson LA, Appel SH (1970) J Neurochem 17: 21-28

20. Karpati G, Carpenter S, Wolfe LS, Andermann F (1977) Neurology 27: 32-42

21. De Leon GA, Kabach MM, Elfenbein IB et al (1969) John Hopkins Med J 125: 205-211

22. Neville BGR, Lake BD, Stephens R et al (1973) Brain 96: 97-120

23. O'Brien JS (1983) In : Stanburry JB, Wyngarden JB, Fredrichson DS et al, eds. The metabolic basis of inherited disease, 5th ed New York : Mac Graw-Hill, 1983, pp 945-969

24. Goldman JE, Katz D, Rapin I et al (1981) Ann Neurol 9: 465-475

25. Suzuki Y, Nakamura N, Fukuoka K et al (1977) Hum Genet 36: 219-229

26. Nakano T, Ikeda S, Kondo K et al (1985) Neurology 35: 875-880

27. Johnson WG (1981) Neurology 31: 1453-1456

28. O'Brien JS (1978) Am J Hum Genet 30: 672-674

29. Suzuki K, Suzuki K, Rapin I (1970) Neurology 20: 190-204

30. Rapin I, Suzuki K, Suzuki K, Valsamis MP (1976) Arch Neurol 33: 120-130

31. Meek D, Wolfe LS, Andermann E, Andermann F (1984) Ann Neurol 15: 348-352

32. Goldie WD, Holzman D, Suzuki K (1977) Ann Neurol 2: 156-158

33. Rapin I, Goldfisher S, Katzman R et al (1978) Ann Neurol 3: 234-242

34. O'Brien JS (1977) Biochem Biophys Res Commun 79: 1136-1141

35. Franceschetti S, Uziel G, Di Donato S et al (1980) J Neurol Neurosurg Psych 43: 934-940

36. Shapira Y, Harel S, Russel A (1977) J Med Sci 13: 161-164

37. Di Mauro S, Bonilla E, Zeviani M et al (1985) Ann Neurol 17: 521-538

38. Linn TC, Pettit FH, Reed LJ (1969) Proc Natl Acad Sci 62: 234-241

39. Blass JP, Avigan J, Uhlendorf BW (1970) J Clin Invest 49: 423-432

40. Blass JP, Schulman JD, Young DS, Hom E (1972) J Clin Invest 51: 1845-1851

41. Prick M, Gabreels F, Renier W et al (1981) Neurology 31: 398-404

42. Pincus JH (1972) Dev Med Child Neurol 14: 87-101

43. Kalimo H, Lundberg PO, Olsson Y (1979) Ann Neurol 6: 200-206

44. Schwartz Wj, Hutchison HT, Berg BO (1981) Ann Neurol 10: 268-271

45. Farmer TW, Veath L, Miller AL et al (1973) Neurology 23: 429 (abst)

46. De Vivo DC, Haymond MW, Obert KA (1979) Ann Neurol 6: 483-494

47. Evans OB (1981) Arch Neurol 38: 515-519

48. Reynolds SF, Blass JP (1976) Neurology 26: 625-628

49. Di Mauro S, Zeviani M, Servidei S et al (1987) Proc NY Acad Sci, in press

50. Di Mauro S, Mendell JR, Sahenk A et al (1980) Neurology 30: 795-804

51. Di Mauro S, Servidei S, Zeviani M et al (1987) Ann Neurol, in press

52. Capaldi RA, Malatesta F, Darley-Usmar VM (1983) Biochim Biphys Acta 726: 135-148

53. Fukuhara N, Tokiguchi S, Shirakawa S, Tsubeki T (1980) J Neurol Sci 47: 117-133

54. Di Mauro S (1987) Personal communication

© 1987 Elsevier Science Publishers B.V. (Biomedical Division)
Extrapyramidal disorders in childhood
L. Angelini et al. editors

IDIOPATHIC AND SYMPTOMATIC DYSTONIAS

LUCIA ANGELINI, VIVIANA RUMI, NARDO NARDOCCI

Department of Child Neurology, Istituto Neurologico "C. Besta", 20133 Milano (Italy)

DEFINITION

Dystonia, derived from the greek δυσ and τονυσ , is the word coined by Oppenheim (1) to signify an alteration of muscle tone without pyramidal deficit.

This faulty muscle tone, generally triggered by voluntary movements, has been described as an irregular involvement of functionally conjugated groups of muscles with coexisting hypotonia and hypertonia. This variability of the muscle tone was typically present in a particular disease characterised by cramps, identified by Schwalbe in 1908 (2). Previously considered as a hysterical symptom, Oppenheim then affirmed its aetiology as organic. He extended the term Dystonia to indicate, not only the faulty tone, but also the abnormal movements and postures peculiar to this pathological condition. He defined this bizarre progressive disease using two different terms: "Dysbasia lordotica progressiva" to underline the worsening of the postures and "Dystonia muscolorum deformans" to focus on the abnormal muscle tone and the fixed ultimate postures. The latter term became accepted in neurological terminology along with its synonym "Torsion Dystonia", introduced by Mendel in 1919 (3). Since then, the term "Dystonia" has signified not only the fluctuation of the tone, as described by Oppenheim, but also a definite neurological disease.

Herz, in 1944 (4), definied the diagnostic criteria of the disease and, on the basis of EMG data, emphasized the simultaneous sustained activation of agonists and antagonists as determining the dystonic movements and postures. The latter have been defined as slow and long sustained.

This definition has been revised and expanded, in 1962, by Denny Brown (5-6), who considered the Dystonia as a fixed or relatively fixed attitude, produced by a sustained muscle contraction.

Marsden (7) finally, in 1982, and Fahn, in 1984, arrived at the definition of Dystonia comprising both postures and movements. This coincided with the Ad hoc Committee's (1984) proposal as follows: "Dystonia is a syndrome of sustained muscle contraction, frequently causing twisting and repetitive movements or abnormal postures" (8). Both dystonic postures and movements can be referred to the same mechanism, that is a sustained muscle contraction combined with subverted reciprocal innervation. When this spasmodic contraction is continuous, it causes a dystonic posture, when it is intermittent it gives rise to a dystonic movement (9). The more frequent dystonic postures are the following.

On the upper extremities: flexion or extension of fingers, inversion of forearms and hands with hyperpronation of wrists.

On the lower extremities: forced plantar flexion of foot rotated inward until equinovarus position, buckling knees.

On the axis: torticollis, retrocollis, tortipelvis and kyphoscoliosis.

The more grotesque postures are those described by Oppenheim as "peacock's trunk" and "dromedary gait" (extreme tortipelvis with backward bending over of the trunk) or appearance of sphinx (in the prone position, when the hyperextension of the head - retrocollis - becomes fixed).

Sleep and general anaesthesia provide a respite, but soft tissue fibrosis and degenerative changes in the joints are finally succeeded by permanent deformities.

Dystonic movements are ubiquitarian, generally slow, long sustained, powerful, usually repetitive, always unpatterned, resembling screw or snake, influenced by the placement of the affected body parts into a specific position, elicited by sensory input and movements, but also spontaneous, increased with fatigue, stress and emotional states, suppressed with relaxation and sleep and characteristically reduced by "sensory tricks" (the resort to tactile or proprioceptive stimuli can often lessen or eliminate severe postures).

Action Dystonia is defined as a superimposition of any involuntary bizarre component on a voluntary movement when motor abnormalities are not yet present during rest (10,11,12).

Dystonic movements, dystonic postures and their combination characterize the Torsion Dystonia in accordance with Zeman and Dyken (13). In this disease, dystonia is usually present continually throughout the day.

When dystonia is intermittent and/or variable, it might be considered a variant form, the "dystonia with marked diurnal fluctuation" by Segawa

(14,15,16).

When dystonia occurs in paroxysmal bursts, followed by a return to normality, without neurological signs between the attacks, it is referred to as paroxysmal dystonia, another variant of Torsion Dystonia (17,18)

CLASSIFICATION

TABLE I
CLASSIFICATION BY DISTRIBUTION

---

1) FOCAL DYSTONIA :   involvement of a single body part:

   - Blepharospasm
   - Oromandibular dystonia
   - Dystonic adductor dysphonia
   - Torticollis
   - Writer's cramp

2) SEGMENTAL DYSTONIA :   involvement of two or more contiguous regions:
   - CRANIAL : two or more parts of cranial or neck musculature are affected;
   - AXIAL   : neck and trunk are affected;
   - BRACHIAL : one arm and axial;
                 both arms ± neck ± trunk;
   - CRURAL   : one leg and trunk;
                 both legs ± trunk.

3) GENERALIZED DYSTONIA :   involvement of multiple parts of the body
                             (segmental crural dystonia and any other segment)

4) MULTIFOCAL DYSTONIA :   involvement of two or more non-contiguous parts.

5) HEMIDYSTONIA   :   involvement of one side of the body

In accordance with Marsden and Fahn (12), Torsion Dystonia can be classified by three criteria: 1) Age at onset, 2) Aetiology, 3) Topography of the abnormal movements.

1) There are three categories: childhood (0-12 years), adolescence (13-20 years), adulthood (> 20 years.)

2) The aetiology divides the dystonia into two groups: Idiopathic (or primary) and Symptomatic (or secondary). The Idiopathic Dystonia is subdivided into

sporadic and familiar.

3) Regarding the bodily distribution Marsden and Harrison (19) proposed a schematic classification in focal, segmental and generalized dystonia. To this, the Ad Hoc Committee (8) added the following, more extensive classification. (Table I).

Idiopathic Dystonia

The patterns of genetic transmission are still incompletely clarified. There are sporadic and familiar Idiopathic Dystonias (20,21,23,24,25,26,10). Among these latter three hereditary patterns, the following are recognized: autosomal dominant transmission, autosomal recessive transmission (prevalent in Ashkenazi Jewish population) and X-linked inheritance (exclusively present in some populations of the Philippines).

The occurrence of the dominant forms, has been established by Zeman and Dyken (13), who detected formes frustes in the families of affected patients. In accordance with Marsden and Fahn (12) the genetic roots of the disease might be revised by the systematic investigation of the families of spy-symptoms such as stuttering, clumsiness and tremor.

The characteristic presenting symptom of Idiopathic Dystonia is action dystonia, i.e. the appearance of abnormal movements during some specific actions, absent at rest and sparing other actions of the same affected part of the body. Since action dystonia primarily affects functions with high significance in interactive relationships as gait and writing, the bizarre motor behavior, then, is often misinterpreted as conversion disorder and treated by psychiatry (27,28).

Subsequently action dystonia can be activated by less specific actions of the affected limb. During further evolution of the disease, actions of other districts of the body can trigger dystonic movements of the affected limb by overflow.

Finally dystonic movements occur also during rest and fixed postures appear. Nevertheless, the patients can, surprisingly, perform skilful movements (Wimmer's kinesia paradoxica) (10).

In addition to the dystonic movements and postures, other movement disorders such as facial grimacing, blepharospasm, tremor and, more seldom, myoclonus can be observed.

To define the latter, Obeso (29) introduced the term of "myoclonic dystonia", although the EMG pattern is characteristic of Dystonia rather than of Myoclonus.

Dysartria, dysphonia (dystonic adductor dyphonia) and dysphagia are other additional symptoms. The variability of muscle tone, of plastic quality at the beginning and springy later, and slight muscle hypertrophy with disarmonic distribution, are further semeiotic findings of the disease.

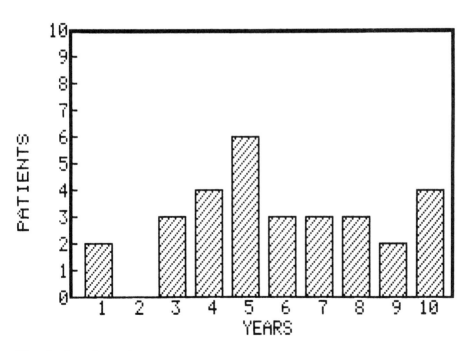

Fig. 1. Age at onset.

In Idiopathic Dystonia there is no pyramidal deficit, no cerebellar signs, no sensory disturbances or cranial nerve defect, no mental deterioration, no personality changes. With regard to pyramidal signs, the striatal foot, as described by Duvoisin (30), can be associated with Hunt's pseudo-Babinski (31), extension of the big toe elicited by cutaneoplantar stimulation and accompanied by an increase of plantar flexion and inward rotation of the foot. The absence of other neurological signs constitutes one of the diagnostic criteria for diagnosis of Idiopathic Torsion Dystonia proposed by Herz and Marsden (4,7).

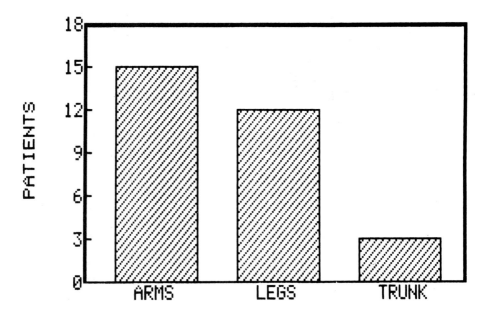

Fig. 2. Site of onset.

The other are the following:

- a disease characterized by the development of dystonic movements and postures;

- no perinatal history, early development normal;

- no history prior to onset of the disease of any known precipitating illness or
  exposure to drugs known to provoke torsion dystonia;

- investigations negative for any cause for the disease.

The disease has different clinical features when the onset is in adulthood or in
childhood.

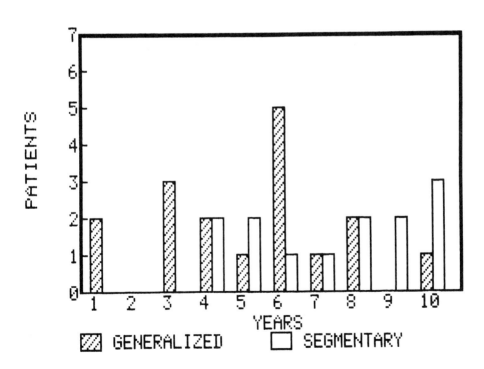

Fig. 3. Age at onset versus generalization.

88

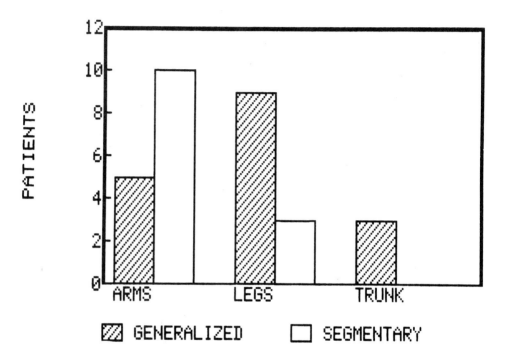

Fig. 4. Site of onset versus generalization.

In the childhood form of the disease, while diagnostic criteria are quite known, the prognostic ones have not yet been defined. In fact all the authors (12,19,32) are acquainted with the more severe progression and the tendency to the generalization of dystonia in childhood, but the course of the disease and the final disability seem to be less known.

Our aim is to contribute to the knowledge of the natural history of Idiopathic dystonia in childhood with our own observations.

30 young patients who attended the Neurological Institute of Milan in the last 15 years are reported; the age at onset of the disease ranges between 1 and 10

years (Fig. 1). The maximum incidence of the onset of the disease is between 5 and 10 years. However, we also have younger patients. With regard to the distribution of the presenting symptom, the axial dystonia is very rare; dystonia always affects the limbs (Fig. 2).

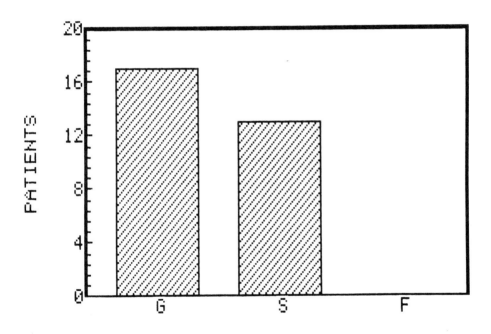

Fig. 5 Course of the disease.
   G = generalized
   S = segmentary
   F = focal

The generalization characterizes the subsequent evolution of the disease in most of the cases. The generalization is more frequent when the onset is early and when the dystonia primarily involves the legs (Fig. 3, 4). Several patients with segmentary dystonia are also present; no focal dystonia has been observed (Fig. 5).

In accordance with the other authors, the additional symptoms are action tremor, facial grimacing and, less frequently, myoclonus. The dysarthria is frequently present; more seldom dysphagia and dysphonia. No mental deterioration has been detected; on the contrary, several patients had and maintained an above-average I.Q. Regarding the intellectual capacities an interesting difference has been observed in the sporadic versus familiar cases. In fact, these latter have a lower I.Q.

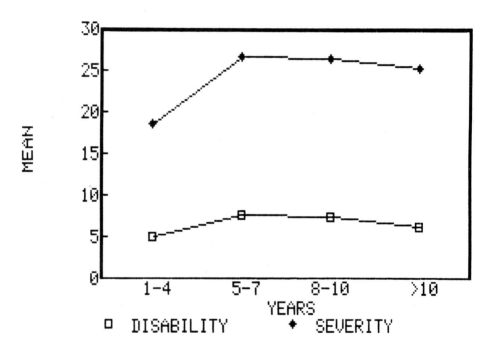

Fig. 6. Course of idiopathic dystonia evaluated by Fahn and Marsden disability and severity rating scales. The evaluations refer to 15 patients, who have been performed at four controls, respectively between 1 to 4 years, 5 to 7 years, 8 to 10 years, > 10 years from the beginning of the disease

The course of the disease in all the patients has been characterized by a fast progression in the first four years of the illness with a subsequent relative stabilization.

Functional disability, evaluated by Fahn and Marsden rating scale (33), is not very severe in our cases, maintaining most of the patients' self care ability (Fig. 6). All these considerations suggest quite a favourable prognosis.

Symptomatic Dystonia

The Symptomatic Dystonias are summarized in the following table (Table II) (34-60).

While Idiopathic Dystonia is exclusively characterized by dystonic symptoms, the presence of other neurological signs is suggestive of a Symptomatic Dystonia. The clinical history and the general examination are indicative of a differential diagnosis. Nevertheless, there are some useful semeiotic criteria (12).

The onset of the Symptomatic Dystonia is never characterized by action dystonia, pathognomonic presenting symptom of Idiopathic Dystonia. Both abnormal movements at rest and fixed postures are present since the onset of the disease. Neither kinesia paradoxica nor sensory tricks, peculiar phenomena in Idiopathic Dystonia, have ever been observed.

Dysarthria and hypophonia (but not dystonic adductor dystonia) are more frequent.

Risus sardonicus and, in accordance with our observations, oromandibular dystonia, never detected in Idiopatic Dystonia, are also frequent.

While Idiopathic Dystonia is slowly and irregularly progressive with plateaus or rarely partial remissions and subsequent recurrence, the progression of Symptomatic Dystonia is faster.

The above description of clinical features in the Symptomatic Dystonia perfectly fits the clinical picture of an homogeneous group of dystonic patients with striatal degeneration visualized by the C.T. scan.

These patients have been observed during the past 15 years in the Neurological Institute of Milan and no similar reports seem to have been reported by other authors.

TABLE II

CLASSIFICATION OF SYMPTOMATIC DYSTONIA

---

1) Associated with other hereditary neurological syndromes:
   - Wilson's disease
   - Huntington's disease
   - Hallervorden-Spatz disease
   - Progressive pallidal degeneration
   - Juvenile neuronal ceroid-lipofuscinosis
   - Metachromatic leukodistrophy
   - GM_1 and GM_2 gangliosidosis
   - Hexosaminidase A and B deficiency
   - Aminoacidopathies and organic acidurias
     (Homocystinuria, glutaric acidaemia, methylmalonic aciduria)
   - Lesch-Nyhan syndrome
   - Ataxia-telangiectasia
   - Leigh's syndrome
   - Infantile bilateral striatal necrosis
   - Dystonic lipidosis (sea-blue histiocytosis)
   - Others (Leber's disease, Joseph's disease, Hartnup's disease, Intraneuronal
     inclusion disease, Familial basal ganglia calcifications, Rett's
     syndrome, Triosephosphate isomerase deficiency)

2) Due to known environmental cause:
   - Perinatal cerebral injury (Athetoid cerebral palsy; Delayed onset dystonia)
   - Encephalitis and postinfections (Reye's syndrome; Subacute sclerosing
     leukoencephalopathy)
   - Head trauma
   - Thalamotomy
   - Brainstem lesion
   - Focal cerebral vascular injury
   - Brain tumor
   - Multiple sclerosis
   - Others (Cervical cord injury; peripheral injury)
   - Drugs (D_2 receptor antagonists; Levodopa; Ergotism; Anti-convulsants)
   - Toxins (Mn - Co - Methanol)
   - Metabolic disorders: hypoparathyroidism

3) Dystonia associated with Parkinsonism

4) Psychogenic dystonia

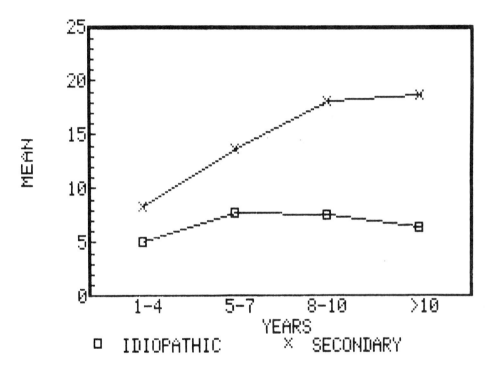

Fig. 7. Disability of Idiopathic and Secondary Dystonia evaluated by Fahn and
Marsden Rating Scale.

In comparison with the group of Idiopathic Dystonia, the Symptomatic Dystonia
group displays a more accelerated progressive course of the disease without
stabilization, a more severe disability (Fig. 7 and 8), presence of pyramidal
signs and a lower I.Q.

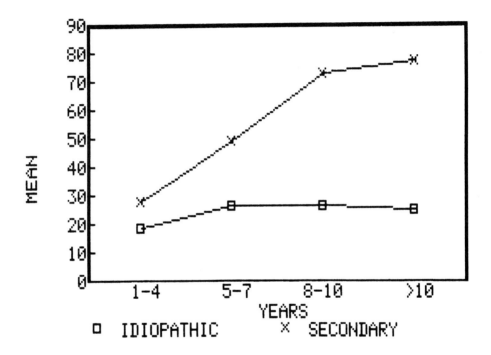

Fig. 8. Severity of Idiopathic and Secondary Dystonia evaluated by Fahn and
Marsden Rating Scale.
   Both evaluations (Fig. 7 and 8) refer to 15 patients with Idiopathic
Dystonia and to 8 patients with Secondary Dystonia, those with the
longer follow-up, and have been performed at four controls, respectively
between 1 to 4 years, 5-7 years, 8-10 years, > 10 years from the
beginning of the disease.

Clinical Investigations.

 The diagnostic approach can be differently codified with regard to Idiopathic and Symptomatic Dystonias as follows (Tables III and IV).

TABLE III

INVESTIGATIONS FOR PATIENTS WITH TYPICAL FEATURES OF IDIOPATHIC DYSTONIA

- Videotape
- Quantitative assessment on Fahn-Marsden rating scales
- CBC - electrolytes - ERS - uric acid
- Lysosomal enzymes on peripheral blood (Arylsuphatase A, β -galactosidase,
  α-N-acetylglucosaminidase)
- Blood and urinary copper - serum ceruloplasmin
- Slitlamp examination
- EEG
- CT scan - MR scan
- I.Q. (WISC)

TABLE IV

INVESTIGATIONS FOR PATIENTS WITH CLINICAL FEATURES ATYPICAL FOR IDIOPATHIC
DYSTONIA

- Videotape
- Quantitative assessment on Fahn-Marsden rating scales
- CBC - electrolytes - ERS - uric acid
- Urinalysis
- Immunoglobulins - alpha-fetoprotein
- Fresh blood smear for acanthocytes
- Lysosomal enzymes on peripheral blood (Arylsulphatase A, β-galactosidase,
  α-N-acetylglucosaminidase)
- Arterial blood pH - lactate - pyruvate
- Electron microscopy of leukocytes and skin and/or conjunctival biopsy
- Urine for mucopolysaccharides and oligosaccharides
- Urine for quantitative organic acids
- Urine for quantitative aminoacids
- EMG - nerve conduction
- Evoked Potentials (PEV - ABR - SEP)
- Electroretinogram
- Nerve and muscle biopsy with electron microscopy (if EMG,VCM,VCS are
  abnormal)
- I.Q. (WISC)

A videotape recording is useful for both Idiopathic and Symptomatic Dystonias,
to evaluate either the course of the disease or a response to pharmacological or
surgical treatment. A quantitative evaluation can be performed by the Fahn and

Marsden rating scales (33).

The severity scale evaluates both the factors which precipitate the dystonic movements (provoking factors) and the severity of the movements in each part of the body.

The functional disability scale evaluates the involvement of functions as: speech, writing, feeding, eating and swallowing, hygiene, dressing and walking.

In cases with history and clinical features typical of idiopathic dystonia, the investigations should be limited mainly to exclude the Wilson's disease and, moreover, some phenotypic variants of delayed onset lysosomal diseases, such as Metachromatic leukodystrophies, GM_1 and GM_2 Gangliosidosis.

CT and MR are necessary to exclude symptomatic dystonias due to lesions of the Basal Ganglia.

Instead, cases with clinical features atypical of idiopathic dystonia, need more complex laboratory work to detect several possible causes of dystonia, as shown in Table II.

CONCLUSIONS

Torsion dystonia is a syndrome which may be classified, in accordance with different aetiology, in primary and secondary forms.

The primary, or idiopathic, torsion dystonia has an unknown biochemical and pathological basis.

With regard to the secondary forms, some recent reports show lesions prevalently in the putamen, suggesting a possible role of this structure in determining dystonia.

Also our dystonic patients with a lesion in the putamen, documented by CT and MR, could confirm this hypothesis.

REFERENCES

1. Oppenheim H (1911) Neurologie Centralblatt, 30, 1090-1107.
2. Schwalbe W (1908) Eine eigentumliche tonische Krampfform mit hysterischen Symptomen. Inaugural Dissertation. G. Schade, Berlin
3. Mendel K (1919) Monatschr Psychiatr Neurol 46: 309-361
4. Herz E (1944) Arch Neurol Psychiatr 51: 20-26
5. Denny Brown D (1962) The basal ganglia and their relation to disorders of movement. Oxford University Press, London

6. Denny Brown D (1962) The Basal ganglia. Oxford University Press, London
7. Marsden CD, Parkes JD, Quinn N (1982) In: Marsden CD, Fahn S (eds) Movement Disorders. Butterworths: London, pp 96-122
8. Ad Hoc Committee (1984) Ad Hoc Committee of the Dystonia Medical Research Foundation met in February 1984.
9. Kanazawa I (1986) In: Vinken PJ, Bruyn GW, Klawans HL (eds) Handbook of Clinical Neurology Vol 5. Elsevier: Amsterdam, pp 65-85
10. Bruyn GW, Roos RAC (1986) In: Vinken PJ, Bruyn GW, Klawans HL (eds) Handbook of Clinical Neurology Vol 5. Elsevier: Amsterdam, pp 519-528
11. Marsden CD (1987) In: Marsden CD, Fahn S (eds) Movement Disorders 2. Butterworths: London, pp 332-358
12. Rothwell JC, Obeso JA (1987) In: Marsden CD, Fahn S (eds) Movement Disorders 2. Butterworths: London, pp 313-331
13. Zeman W, Dyken P (1968) Neurology 10: 517-543
14. Segawa M, Osaka A, Miyagawa F, Nomura Y, Imai H (1976) Adv. Neurol. 14: 215-233
15. Sunohara N, Mano Y, Ando K, Satoyoshi E (1985) Ann. Neurol 17: 39-45
16. Ouvrier RA (1978) Ann Neurol 4: 412-417
17. Fahn S, Bressman S (1983) Neurology 33 Suppl. 2: 131
18. Lance JW (1977) Ann Neurol 2: 285-293
19. Marsden CD, Harrison MJG, Budney S (1976) Adv Neurol 14: 177-187
20. Cooper IS, Cullinan T, Riklan M (1976) Adv Neurol 14: 157-169
21. Eldridge R, Gottlieb R (1976) Adv Neurol 14: 457-474
22. Lee LV, Pascasio FM, Fuentes FD, Viterbo GH (1976) Adv Neurol 14: 137-151
23. Zeman W (1976) Adv Neurol 14: 91-103
24. Eldridge R (1981) Ann Neurol 10: 203-204
25. Burke RE, Fahn S, Brin MF, Bressman S, Moskowitz C (1985) Neurology 35 Suppl 1: 273
26. Nygaard TG, Duvoisin RC (1986) Neurology 36: 1424-1428
27. Fahn S, Williams D, Reches A, Lesser RP, Jankovic C, Silberstein SD (1983) Neurology 33 Suppl 2: 161
28. Lesser RP, Fahn S (1978) Am J Psychiatry 153: 349-452
29. Obeso JA, Rothwell JC, Lang AE, Marsden CD (1983) Neurology 33: 825-830
30. Duvoisin RC, Yahr MD, Lieberman J, Autunes J, Rhee S (1972) Trans Am Neurol Assoc 97: 267
31. Hunt JR (1917) Brain 40: 58-148
32. Marsden CD, Harrison MJG (1947) Brain 97: 793-810
33. Burke RE, Fahn S, Marsden CD, Bressman SB, Moskowitz C, Friedman J (1985) Neurology 35. 73-77
34. De Leon GA, Karback MM, Elfenbein IB, Percy AK, Brady RO (1969) John Hopkins Med J 125: 62-77
35. Gilman S, Barrett RE (1973) J Neurol Sci 19: 189-205
36. Backman DS, Lao-Velez C, Estanol B (1976) Arch Neurol 33: 590
37. Tahmoush AJ, Alpers DH, Feigin RD, Armbrustmacher V, Prensky AL (1976) Arch Neurol 33: 797-807
38. Goldie WD, Holtzman D, Suzuki K (1977) Ann Neurol 2: 156-158
39. Brun A, Killerman M (1979) Eur J Pediat 131: 93-104
40. Crosley CJ, Swender PT (1979) Pediatrics 63: 612-615
41. Bodensteiner JB, Goldblum RM, Goldman AS (1980) Arch Neurol 37: 464-465
42. Burke RE, Fahn S, Gold AP (1980) J Neurol Neurosurg Psychiatry 43: 789-797

98

43. Leibel RL, Shih VE, Goodmand SI, Bauman ML, McCabe ERB, Zwerdling RG (1980) Neurolog! 30: 1163-1168
44. Brett EM, Sheehy MP, Marsden CD (1981) J Neurol Neurosurg Psychiatry 44: 460
45. Goldman JE, Katz D, Rapin I, Purpura DP, Suzuki K (1981) Ann Neurol 9: 465-475
46. Goutieres F, Aicardi J (1982) Ann Neurol 12: 328-332
47. Grimes JD, Hassan MH, Quarrington AM, D'Alton J (1982) Neurology 32: 1033-1035
48. Heath PD, Nightingale S (1982) Ann Neurol 12: 494-495
49. Watts RWE, Spellacy E, Gibbs DA, Allsop J, McKeran RO, Slavin GE (1982) Q J Med 201: 43-78
50. Davous P, Rondot P (1983) J Neurol Neurosurg Psychiatry 46: 283
51. Demierre B, Rondot P (1983) J Neurol Neurosurg Psychiatry 46: 404-409
52. Meek D, Wolfe LS Andermann E, Andermann F (1984) Ann Neurol 15: 348-352
53. Narbona J, Obeso JA, Tunon T, Martinez-Lage JM, Marsden CD (1984) J Neurol Neurosurg Psychiatry 47: 704-709
54. Philippart M, Brown WJ (1984) Ann Neurol 16: 387
55. Lang AE, Clarke JTR, Resch L, Strasberg P, Skomoroski MA, O'Connor P (1985) Neurology 35 Suppl 1: 194
56. Larsen TA, Dunn HG, Jan JE, Calne DB (1985) Neurology 35: 533-537
57. Marsden CD, Obeso JA, Zarranz JJ, Lang AE (1985) Brain 108: 461-483
58. Pettigrew LC, Jankovic J (1985) J Neurol Neurosurg Psychiatry 48: 650-657
59. Novotny EJ Jr, Singh G, Wallace DC, Dorfmann LJ, Louis A, Sogg RL (1986) Neurology 36: 1053.1060
60. Roos RAC, Bruyn GW (1986) In: Vinken PJ, Bruyn GW, Klavans HL (eds) Handbook of Clinical Neurology Vol 5. Elsevier, Amsterdam, pp 541-547

© 1987 Elsevier Science Publishers B.V. (Biomedical Division)
Extrapyramidal disorders in childhood
L. Angelini et al. editors

MYOCLONUS: NOSOLOGICAL AND CLINICAL ASPECTS IN INFANTS AND CHILDREN

JEAN AICARDI

Institut National de la Santé et de la Recherche Médicale and Neurological Unit, Hôpital des Enfants Malades, 149 rue de Sèvres, 75743 Paris Cedex 15 (France)

INTRODUCTION

Myoclonus is a type of involuntary movements that consists of sudden, brief, shocklike muscle contractions arising from the central nervous system and which may be generalized or confined to one or more individual muscle or group of muscles (1,2). This definition excludes muscle fasciculations, myokymias or twitches due to lesions of the lower motor neuron even though they may be phenomenologically similar to myoclonic jerks. The jerks observed in the course of subacute sclerosing panencephalitis are generally regarded as myoclonic (2) although most of them are long-lasting complex involuntary movements that do not have the shock-like brevity of myoclonic jerks. On the other hand, the so-called nocturnal myoclonus (essential) is generally excluded from the group of myoclonic jerks because of the long duration of abnormal movements. The definition of myoclonus does not imply the involvement of any specific anatomical or physiological system or circuit and the understanding of its mechanisms is far from complete. Myoclonus can be produced by cortical, subcortical, brainstem or spinal lesions or it may result from metabolic disturbances without morphologically recognizable brain damage. From a neurophysiological viewpoint it is customary to separate pyramidal myoclonus in which the muscle jerk follows a cortical discharge with a fixed latency that corresponds to the conduction time through the pyramidal tract from the cortex to the affected muscle and extrapyramidal myoclonus in which the pyramidal tract is not involved, the discharge propagating along different pathways (4). Hallett et al (5) recognized several types of reflex myoclonus. In cortical reflex myoclonus, the myoclonic activity is preceded by a cortical spike that may be recorded on the EEG either directly or by back-averaging from the muscle spike and bursts of impulses are propagated downward from the cortex in response to normal afferent volleys. In reticular reflex myoclonus the volleys appear to originate from

the lower brainstem reticular substance and are propagated both
upwards to the upper brainstem and the cortex and downwards along
the spinal cord as shown by the pattern of muscle activation, the
sternomastoid being activated before the facial and limb musculature (6). In ballistic movement overflow myoclonus bursts are only
associated with voluntary rapid movements (7).

Although there may be some correspondence between the neurophysiological mechanism and the cause of myoclonus (e.g. ballistic
overflow myoclonus is a form of essential myoclonus), the same
cause can produce myoclonus through different mechanisms (e.g.
post-hypoxic myoclonus may be of the cortical or reticular reflex
types) and the precise mechanism is often undetermined. As a
result, the most useful classifications are based on clinical features and etiology rather than mechanism (1).

CLINICAL FEATURES AND DIFFERENTIAL DIAGNOSIS

Myoclonus presents itself in various patterns depending on the
distribution, regularity, sensitivity to stimuli and intensity of
the jerks. The amplitude of myoclonic jerks can range from small
contractions that do not result in movement of joints to gross
contractions capable of moving one or several limbs, the trunk
or head, and to provoke falls. The myoclonus can be localized to
a single muscle group, to one limb or segment of limb or it may
involve multiple regions of the body bilaterally including the
axial musculature (generalized or massive myoclonus). When bilateral, the myoclonus can be symmetrical or asymmetrical. Generalized myoclonus is often synchronized, all involved muscles jerking within milliseconds of each other. However, erratic asynchronous jerks of relatively small amplitude may also occur (1,2).
Rhythmic myoclonus is rather uncommon and is usually, but not
always (1), associated with a lesion of brainstem or spinal cord.
Arrhythmic myoclonus, whether massive or localized is more common.
The sensitivity of myoclonus to stimuli is an important character.
Sensory stimuli include light, especially intermittent flashes,
nociceptive events, proprioceptive volleys, e.g. tapping deep
tendon reflexes, muscle stretch or noise. They are mainly effective when they are suddenly applied. Movement is a frequent trigger of myoclonic jerks, especially intentional movement, and the
myoclonus is most marked when attempting to perform a fine motor

task such as reaching for a target. Even the intention of accomplishing a voluntary movement or merely thinking of movement may provoke the jerks, hence the term of action and intention myoclonus applied to such cases (8). In some patients, passive movement can also trigger myoclonic jerks (2). Movement-induced myoclonus may be localized to the segment or limb involved in the actual movement or it may extend to other segments and become generalized even for attempted minimal movements. In rare patients only ballistic movements will induce myoclonus (7).

The differential diagnosis of myoclonus can be difficult. Dystonic movements are clearly different from myoclonic jerks but both types can be associated in some patients (1,9). Muscle fasciculations can be indistinguishable from small amplitude myoclonic jerks and lesions of peripheral nerves or plexus may produce myoclonus-like movements, even though the mechanism remains obscure. Myokymias differ from myoclonus by their wave-like character. The tremor (sometimes called minipolymyoclonus) observed in patients with chronic anterior horn cell disease (10,11) is of small amplitude and irregular but its occurrence with movement can simulate action myoclonus. Choreic movements and tics differ from myoclonic jerks by their resemblance to normal, if purposeless, voluntary movements and longer duration (1,10). However, sudden, brief jerks can occur both in choreas and in Tourette syndrome but other motor activity permits differentiation. Localized epileptic clonias, especially epilepsia partialis continua, are sometimes included in myoclonus (1,2). They are usually increased by voluntary movements. The clinical context, however, is quite different and this type of myoclonus will not be dealt with in this chapter. Startle is also regarded by some authorities as a form of myoclonus (2,12). It is a physiological reaction to sudden stimuli but it may be pathologically increased in hyperekplexia (12) which resembles massive myoclonus. The syndrome of benign infantile myoclonus (13) refers to abnormal movements generally with flexion of the head and trunk sometimes with abduction and flexion of the arms that occur in series in infants 4-12 months of age. These resemble infantile spasms but psychomotor development and EEG tracings remain normal and the course is spontaneously favorable. It seems likely from polygraphic and video recordings that such movements that occur only in awake infants are tics

rather than myoclonias. Asterixis is characterized by sudden loss
of muscle tone in one, or several segments, and results in movements that may be difficult to differentiate from myoclonic jerks
without electrophysiological studies. These show the disappearance
of basal tonic electrical activity in affected muscles without
action potentials (14). Indeed, an interruption of elctromyogra-
phic activity is regularly observed following myoclonic bursts
(15) and may be responsible for part of the clinical manifestations of myoclonus, especially falls (16). Some investigators
consider asterixis as a special form of "negative myoclonus" (14).

ETIOLOGY OF MYOCLONUS IN CHILDREN

Epileptic versus non epileptic myoclonus

   Certain types of myoclonus have a close relationship to epilepsy.
There is no universal agreement, however, as to which types of
myoclonus should be regarded as epileptic. Kelly et al (17) termed
"epileptic" all cases of myoclonus that occurred in patients who
were also subject to nonmyoclonic seizures or had spike or spike-
wave discharges in their EEGs, and "nonepileptic" other cases.
Marsden et al (1) limited the group of epileptic myoclonus to
cases in which seizures dominate and there is no encephalopathy,
at least initially. They termed symptomatic those cases in which
progressive or static encephalopathy dominates (table 1).

   The group of epileptic myoclonus, as defined by these authors,
includes epileptic syndromes, such as West syndrome and Lennox-
Gastaut syndrome, in which the brief ictal events observed are
more often short tonic or atonic seizures than true myoclonus.
They involve sustained, even if short-lasting, muscle contractions rather than shock-like movements. It is however customary
to include these syndromes in the group of the myoclonic epilepsies
(32).

   The group of symptomatic myoclonus in Marsden's classification
includes a large number of heterogeneous conditions, many of which
also feature epileptic seizures in addition to myoclonic jerks.
In some of these, myoclonus is a major manifestation whereas in
others it is only an occasional component of the clinical picture.
Thus, post anoxic encephalopathy or renal failure are consistently
marked by intense myoclonic activity whilst myoclonus is only
rarely seen in the course of spinocerebellar degenerations or
of the basal ganglia.

TABLE I

CLASSIFICATION OF MYOCLONUS (MODIFIED FROM MARSDEN ET AL 1)

1 Physiologic myoclonus (normal subjects)
2 Essential myoclonus (no known cause and no other gross
  neurological deficit)
    - Hereditary (autosomal dominant)
    - Sporadic
3 Epileptic myoclonus (nonprogressive myoclonic epilepsies)
    - Infantile spasms*
    - Lennox-Gastaut syndrome*
    - Cryptogenetic myoclonic epilepsies (early and late types)
    - Myoclonic (clonic) absences
    - Juvenile myoclonic epilepsy (Janz syndrome)
    - Photomyoclonic seizures
4 Symptomatic myoclonus (progressive encephalopathies including
  the progressive myoclonic epilepsies)
    - Metabolic (e.g. uremia, dialysis syndrome, hepatic failure)
    - Toxic (bismuth, methylbromide, DDT, piperazines, heavy
      metals, poisoning, levodopa, penicillin, other drugs)
    - Physical encephalopathies (post-hypoxia, post-traumatic,
      heat stroke, electric shock, decompression injury)
    - Viral encephalopathies (subacute panencephalitis, encepha-
      litis lethargica, other encephalitides, infantile myoclonic
      encephalopathy of Kinsbourne, Creutzfeld-Jakob disease)
    - Storage diseases (see table II)
    - Spinocerebellar degenerations
    - Basal ganglia degenerations

* Usually included among the myoclonic epilepsy despite the fact
  that jerks are more sustained and of longer duration than classical myoclonic jerks.

Such separation is somewhat artificial. For example, Baltic
myoclonus and Lafora disease belong to separate groups even though
they may be quite difficult to distinguish clinically at onset
and both have prominent epileptic (nonmyoclonic) seizures. Other
investigators (2,10) consider "epileptic" the myoclonic jerks,
usually of the massive type, which are associated with spike-wave
bursts on the EEG and as "nonepileptic" those jerks that are unas-
sociated with paroxysmal EEG events and are mostly of the erratic
type. Such a separation is far from absolute. Erratic, multifocal
myoclonic jerks are frequently seen in patients with the Lennox-
Gastaut syndrome or with early myoclonic epilepsies, and massive
myoclonic jerks with and without associated spike-wave bursts may
occur in the same patient even on the same EEG record (18). In
this paper, a classification derived from that of Marsden will be
used. However, progressive "degenerative" myoclonic epilepsies
including the Baltic type will be studied with symptomatic myoclonus. The group of the myoclonic epilepsies which has been reviewed in detail previously (19) will not be further considered.

Etiology of Myoclonus outside the group of the myoclonic Epilepsies
    The age and mode of onset, the family history as well as the
natural history of the myoclonus and of associated manifestations
form the basis for clinical diagnosis.
    Physiologic myoclonus occurs in normal children and does not
usually pose diagnostic problems. Hypnagogic jerks are common in
older children and adolescents (20) and fragmentary myoclonias
are seen during deep sleep and especially during stage I sleep
and REM sleep (2).
    In a few neonates, clonic jerks occur repetitively in series
that may last minutes to hours during deep sleep and can be mis-
taken for epileptic seizures (21). However, neurological examination is normal, there are no EEG abnormalities even during
attacks and this benign neonatal sleep myoclonus spontaneously
subsides in a few weeks or months.
    Essential myoclonus is a disorder in which myoclonus occurs as
the sole neurological abnormality and etiology is unknown (1).
The myoclonus is usually arrhythmic and diffusely distributed,
but all types can be observed. Action myoclonus has been reported
(15). The condition can be either familial (usually with dominant

transmission) or sporadic (22). Tremor may alternate with myoclonus within the same lineage (23). The disease usually has its
onset after 5-7 years of age. It is not progressive and can be
improved by drug treatment (clonazepam).

Symptomatic myoclonus. A host of CNS disorders include myoclonus
amongst their manifestations (table II). Myoclonus can have a
sudden or rapid onset or develop in a progressive manner.

Myoclonus of sudden or rapid onset includes myoclonus resulting
from exogenous intoxication, e.g. by DDT and methylbromide or by
a number of drugs notably piperazine anthelminthic medications
and levodopa (24), as well as from endogenous toxicity. The latter includes some cases of hepatic failure and, especially, uremia
(2) and dialysis encephalopathy (25). Post-anoxic myoclonus usually
appears following cardiac arrest and resuscitation. It is commonly
an action and intention myoclonus (15) and may respond to serotonin precursors. Myoclonus has also been reported following heat
stroke, head trauma and electric shock. The circumstances of appearance of the myoclonic jerks in such cases render the diagnosis
easy.

Myoclonus constitutes the main manifestation of the clonic encephalopathy of Kinsbourne (26). The condition affects primarily
children under 2 years of age. It is marked by the sudden onset
of intense myoclonus of the trunk and limbs associated with chaotic oscillations of the eyeballs in all directions (opsoclonus).
The EEG is normal or displays mild nonspecific abnormalities. Both
the jerks and the eye movements tend to decrease slowly but may
recur for years with intervening infections. The syndrome is
usually of unknown cause. It may uncommonly be the first manifestation of a ganglioneuroblastoma (27), especially when the tumor
is located in the thorax. A similar syndrome with a more acute
course and with pleocytosis of the CSF may be seen with demonstrated enteroviral infections (28). Myoclonus is a hallmark of
the subacute spongiform encephalopathies but these are not observed in children. As indicated earlier, the jerks of subacute panencephalitis may represent true myoclonias (2). In the neonate,
erratic myoclonus with onset within 24 to 72 hours of birth, associated with profound hypotonia and a suppression-burst pattern
on the EEG, suggests the diagnosis of nonketotic hyperglycinemia
(29) or, very rarely of D-glyceric acidemia.

TABLE II

MAIN CAUSES OF CHRONIC PROGRESSIVE MYOCLONUS

Group I : Typical progressive myoclonus epilepsy
- Lafora body disease
- Progressive myoclonic epilepsy "degenerative" types (including "Baltic" myoclonic epilepsy)
- Dyssynergia cerebellaris myoclonica (Ramsay Hunt syndrome)
- Juvenile neuronopathic Gaucher's disease (type III)
- Sialidosis type I (cherry-red spot-myoclonus syndrome) ; type II (galactosialidosis) ; mucolipidosis type I
- Myoclonic epilepsy with ragged-red fibers (MERRF)
- Juvenile neuroaxonal dystrophy
- Myoclonic epilepsy with renal failure

Group II : Atypical progressive myoclonic epilepsy
- Neuronal ceroid-lipofuscinosis
    early infantile type (Santavuori-Hagberg)
    late infantile type (Jansky-Bielschowsky)
    early juvenile type (Cavanagh)
    juvenile type (Spielmeyer-Vogt)
- Nonspecific poliodystrophies
    Alpers disease
    poliodystrophies with hepatic failure (at times with lactic acidosis)
- Hexosaminidase deficiency
    Tay-Sachs disease
    Sandhoff disease
    A B variant
- Wilson's disease
- Huntington's chorea (myoclonic variant)
- Hallervorden-Spatz disease
- Dystonia musculorum deformans
- Dentatorubral-pallidoluysian atrophy
- Biopterin deficiency
- Biotin-dependency and biotinidase deficiency

Myoclonus of progressive onset can result from a large number of degenerative disorders of the CNS which feature myoclonias as

one of their major manifestations. Some of them fit the clinical
picture of progressive myoclonus epilepsy according to the description of Unverricht and Lundborg. In a majority of the cases, however, the disorders of this group have relatively characteristic
clinical, EEG and other features that permit recognition, and
enzymatic assays or peripheral tissue biopsies are available to
confirm their diagnosis (30). The main conditions that give rise
to progressive myoclonic encephalopathies -often in association
with epileptic seizures- are listed in table II. The disorders
have been divided into two groups. The first group includes those
disorders that produce the "classical" picture of progressive myoclonus epilepsy (31,32). The second group comprises those conditions in which the myoclonic jerks are not the most prominent feature -even at onset of the disease- but only one part of a complex
neurological picture in which other signs may well overshadow the
myoclonus. Only some salient features of the most important conditions listed will be reviewed.

Lafora body disease (33,34) is an autosomal recessive disorder
that begins between 10 and 18 years of age by generalized tonic-
clonic seizures. Partial seizures, however, are common and especially affect the visual cortex (30). The myoclonic jerks appear
later. They are usually of the erratic type, of small amplitude
and often do not produce movements of the joints. The jerks are
asynchronous, arrhythmic and usually occur spontaneously. They
are often increased by stimuli such as intermittent light, touch
or attempted movement. Mental deterioration progresses rapidly.
The EEG initially shows only spike-wave complexes on light stimulation but basal rhythm rapidly deteriorates. Diagnosis can be
confirmed by skin, muscle or hepatic biopsy showing the typical
polyglucosan bodies. The picture of the so-called *degenerative
types of progressive myoclonus epilepsy* is initially indistinguishable from that of Lafora disease apart from an earlier age of
onset (7-12 years). The myoclonus is often more prominent than in
Lafora body disease and is commonly very sensitive to stimuli
especially attempted movement. Mental deterioration, if any, is
very slow. Cerebellar signs are usually present but may be difficult to evidence because of the movement-induced myoclonus.
Contrary to Lafora disease, there is no specific pathology but
only degenerative lesions of the Purkinje cells and, in many cases,

of the dentate nucleus and olivary body, and the diagnosis rests
entirely on clinical grounds (35). Most cases seem to be transmitted in an autosomal recessive manner. The EEG shows variable
degrees of abnormality : in all patients, photic stimulation
induces spike-wave bursts that may also occur spontaneously and
are often associated clinically with massive myoclonic jerks. The
background rhythms are variably affected. In the so-called Baltic
type, which is particularly frequent in Finland (36), slowing of
the tracings seems to be an early feature. In other types, the
background EEG remains normal for years, apart from the occurrence
of paroxysms. Roger et al (37) set apart *the Ramsay-Hunt syndrome*
in which the EEG is similar to that of primary generalized epilepsy and the myoclonus is essentially movement induced. In most
cases, massive myoclonic jerks, of the type observed in juvenile
myoclonic epilepsy are also present. There is probably more than
one type of degenerative myoclonus epilepsy and the exact definition of the various conditions will have to await discovery of
biological markers. A picture virtually identical to that of the
Ramsay Hunt syndrome is produced by *type I sialidosis* which can be
diagnosed by demonstrating the deficit in neuraminidase. Mucolipidosis type I and gangliosialidosis or type II sialidosis are
related disorders in which a short stature and dysmorphic features
reminiscent of those observed in the mucopolysaccharidoses are
present in addition to the myoclonus and the cherry-red spot characteristic of sialidosis type I (38,39). *Juvenile neuropathic
Gaucher* disease can also be the cause of a picture of progressive
myoclonus with or without generalized (30) seizures and often with
supra-nuclear gaze palsies.

Juvenile neuroaxonal dystrophy is also responsible for a progressive myoclonic disease with retinal degeneration (40). Spheroids
can be found in skin or conjunctival biopsy.

A picture closely resembling the Ramsay Hunt syndrome may be
observed in the so-called *myoclonic epilepsy with ragged-red fibers
(MERRF)*, a type of mitochondrial encephalomyopathy (41,42). The
myoclonus is generally of the action and intention type and is
often associated with massive myoclonic jerks and with other types
of seizures. Deafness, a small stature and slow mental deterioration are frequent.

Myoclonic epilepsy and renal failure has been reported from Quebec (43). The myoclonus is also of the action and intention type.

Among the second group of CNS degenerative diseases with myoclonus, the *neuronal ceroid-lipofuscinoses* are the most common condition. In the early infantile type (44) massive myoclonias are a relatively late manifestation. In the late infantile type (Jansky-Bielschowsky), myoclonus is an early and prominent feature (45). Both massive jerks and erratic myoclonias can occur and falls are common. The EEG is very abnormal with slow waves and multifocal spikes. The response to intermittent photic stimulation is distinctive with spike-waves complexes induced over the occipital regions by each flash at rhythms of 1 to 3 per second (46). These represent giant evoked potentials. The course of the disease is rapidly downhill with the appearance of extrapyramidal, pyramidal and cerebellar signs. In the juvenile type (Spielmeyer-Vogt), myoclonus usually follows a protracted period of deteriorating vision, behavioral disturbances and speech difficulties. The myoclonus seems to be mostly of the erratic type (30). In all three types, the EEG is precociously abnormal and convulsive seizures of several types are commonly associated. The diagnosis of ceroid-lipofuscinosis can usually be confirmed by skin or conjunctival biopsy or by electron microscopic study of lymphocytes (47), showing the characteristic lysosomal inclusions.

Nonspecific degeneration of the grey matter (so-called Alpers disease) gives rise to both generalized or partial seizures and to myoclonic jerks, massive or erratic (48). In some cases hepatic dysfunction and, ultimately, hepatic failure occur (49). In some cases abnormal mitochondria have been demonstrated (50).

Myoclonus also occurs in some cases of Wilson's disease, in Hallervorden-Spatz disease, in some cases of dystonia musculorum deformans (myoclonic dystonia) (9) and in Huntington chorea. In the latter condition, it may occasionally be a prominent feature (the myoclonic form) (51). In *Tay-Sachs and Sandhoff diseases* acoustic startles are usually the earliest manifestation. Some investigators include them in the category of myoclonus (2,30). Biotin deficiency has been recently reported in rare patients with intense myoclonic jerking (52) and myoclonus may be a feature of biopterin deficiency (53). Other entities such as dentatorubral-pallidoluysan atrophy (54) and other rares types (55) have not been reported in children.

Only rarely is *rhythmic myoclonus* , especially palatal myoclonus observed in children. I recently saw a child who developed palatal myoclonus during the course of an obscure degenerative CNS disorder. A few similar cases have been reported in adults (56). A benign form of palatal myoclonus without any associated neurological dysfunction and with a self-limited benign course also occurs in children (57). Its mechanism is not understood.

CONCLUSION

The limits of myoclonus are difficult to define precisely even from a phenomenological point of view. There is no pathological change that can be demonstrated consistently in all types and no single neurophysiological mechanism appears to be at play. Despite these difficulties, myoclonus is an important clue to the diagnosis of many CNS disorders. In addition, the introduction of serotonin precursors, clonazepam,and sodium valproate have greatly improved the outlook for patients afflicted with several forms of myoclonus.

REFERENCES

1. Marsden CD, Hallett M, Fahn S (1982) In : Marsden CD, Fahn S (eds) Movement Disorders. Butterworth, London, pp 196-248

2. Gastaut H (1968) Rev Neurol (Paris) 119:1-30

3. Lugaresi E, Cirignotta , Coccagna G, Montana P (1986) In : Fahn S, Marsden CD, Van Woert M (eds) Adv Neurol vol 43. Raven Press, New York, pp 295-307

4. Halliday AM (1967) Brain 90:241-284

5. Hallett M, Chadwick D, Marsden CD (1979) Neurology 29:1107-1125

6. Hallett M, Chadwick D, Adam J, Marsden CD (1977) Arch Neurol 40:253-264

7. Hallett M, Chadwick D, Marsden CD (1977) Brain 100:299-312

8. Lance JW (1986) In : Fahn S, Marsden CD, Van Woert M (eds) Adv Neurol vol 43, Myoclonus, Raven Press, New York,pp 33-55

9. Obeso JA, Rothwell JC, Lang AE, Marsden CD (1983) Neurology 33:825-830

10. Bonduelle M (1968) In : Vinken PJ, Bruyn GW (eds) Handbook of Clinical Neurology vol 6 Diseases of the Basal Ganglia, North Holland, Amsterdam, pp 761-781

11. Spiro AJ (1970) Neurology 20:1124-1126

12. Andermann F, Andermann E (1986) In : Fahn S, Marsden CD, Van Woert M (eds) Adv Neurol vol 43 Myoclonus. Raven Press, New York, pp 321-355

13. Lombroso CT, Fejerman N (1977) Ann Neurol 1:138-143

14. Young RR, Shahani BT (1986) In : Fahn S, Marsden CD, Van Woert M (eds) Adv Neurol vol 43, Myoclonus, Raven Press, New York, pp 137-156

15. Lance JW, Adams RD (1963) Brain 86:111-136

16. Tassinari CA, Lyagoubi S, Santos V, Gambarelli F, Roger J, Dravet C, Gastaut H (1969) Rev Neurol 121:379-383

17. Kelly JJ, Sharbrough FW, Daube JR (1981) Neurology 31:581-589

18. Dravet C, Roger J, Bureau M, Dalla Bernardina B (1982) In : Akimoto H, Kazamatsuri H, Seine M, Ward A (eds) Advances in Epileptology : XIIth Epilepsy International Symposium, Raven Press, New York, pp 135-140

19. Aicardi J (1986) In : Fahn S, Marsden CD, Van Woert M (eds) Adv Neurol vol 43, Myoclonus, Raven Press, New York, pp 11-31

20. Oswald I (1959) Brain 82:92-103

21. Coulter DL, Allen RJ (1982) Arch Neurol 39:191-192

22. Bressman S, Fahn S (1986) In : Fahn S, Marsden CD, Van Woert M (eds) Adv Neurol vol 43, Myoclonus, Raven Press, New York, pp 287-294

23. Korten JJ, Notermans SLH, Frenken CWGM, Gabreels FJM, Joostens EMG (1974) Brain 97:131-138

24. Klawans HL, Carvey PM, Tanner CM, Goetz CG (1986) In : Fahn S, Marsden CD, Van Woert M (eds) Adv Neurol vol 43, Myoclonus, Raven Press, New York, pp 251-264

25. Alfrey AC, Legendre GR, Kachny WD (1976) N Engl J Med 294: 184-188

26. Kinsbourne M (1962) J Neurol Neurosurg Psychiatr 25:271-279

27. Moe PG, Nellhaus G (1970) Neurology 20:756-764

28. Kuban KC, Ephros MA, Freeman RL, Laffell LB, Bresnan MJ (1983) Ann Neurol 13:69-71

29. Dalla Bernardina B, Aicardi J, Goutières F, Plouin P (1979) Neuropaediatrics 10:209-225

30. Rapin I (1986) In : Fahn S, Marsden CD, Van Woert M (eds) Adv Neurol vol 43, Myoclonus, Raven Press, New York, pp 65-85

31. Diebold K (1973) Der erblichen myoklonisch-epileptisch dementiellen Kern syndrome, Springer, Berlin

32. Aicardi J (1986) Epilepsy in children Raven Press, New York

33. Roger J, Gastaut H, Toga M, Soulayrol R, Riges H et al (1965) Rev Neurol, Paris 112:50-61

34. Van Heycop Ten Ham WG, Dejager H (1963) Epilepsia 4:95-119

35. Matthews WB, Howell DA, Stevens DI (1969) J Neurol Neurosurg Psychiatr 32:116-122

36. Koskiniemi M, Donner M, Majuri H, Haltia M, Norio R (1974) Acta Neurol Scand 50:307-332

37. Roger J, Soulayrol R, Hassoun J (1968) Rev Neurol (Paris) 119:85-106

38. Rapin I, Goldfisher S, Katzman R, Engel JJr, O'Brien JS (1978) Ann Neurol 3:234-242

39. Suzuki Y, Nakamura N, Shimada Y, Yotsumoto H, Endo H, Nagashima K (1977) Arch Neurol 34:157-161

40. Scheithauer BW, Forno LS, Dorfman LJ, Kane CA (1978) J Neurol Sci 36:247-258

41. Fukuhara N, Tokiguchi S, Shirakawa K, Tsubaki T (1980) J Neurol Sci 47:117-133

42. Garcia Silva MT, Aicardi J, Goutières F, Chevrie JJ (1987) Neuropediatrics, in press

43. Andermann E, Andermann F, Carpenter S, Wolfe L, Nelson R, Patry G, Boileau J (1986) In : Fahn S, Marsden CD, Van Woert M (eds) Adv Neurol vol 43, Myoclonus, Raven Press, New York, pp 87-103

44. Santavuori P, Haltia M, Rapola J, Raitta C (1973) J Neurol Sci 18:257-267

45. Pampiglione G, Harden A (1973) J Neurol Neurosurg Psychiatr 36:68-74

46. Green JB (1971) Dev Med Child Neurol 13:477-489

47. Arsenio-Nunes ML, Goutières F, Aicardi J (1981) Ann Neurol 9:163-173

48. Adams RD, Lyon G (1982) Hemisphere, Washington, pp 157-158

49. Harding BN, Egger J, Portmann B, Erdohazi M (1986) Brain 109:181-206

50. Prick MJJ, Gabreels FJM, Trijbels JMF (1983) Clin Neurol Neurosurg 85:57-70

51. Garrel S, Joannard A, Feuerstein C, Serre F (1978) Rev Electro-encephalogr Neurophysiol Clin 8:123-128

52. Bressman S, Fahn S, Eisenberg M, Brin M, Maltese W (1986) In : Fahn S, Marsden CD, Van Woert M (eds) Adv Neurol vol 43, Myoclonus, Raven Press, New York, pp 119-125

53. Rey F, Harpey JP, Leeming RJ, Blair JA, Aicardi J, Rey J (1977) Arch Franç Pediatr 34:suppl 2,109-120

54. Naito H, Oyanagi S (1982) Neurology 32:798-807

55. Logigian EL, Kolodny EH, Griffith JF, Filipek PA, Richardson EP Jr (1986) Brain 109:411-429

56. Sperling MR, Herrmann C (1985) Neurology 35:1212-1214

57. Boulloche J, Aicardi J (1984) Arch Fr Pediatr 41:645-647

© 1987 Elsevier Science Publishers B.V. (Biomedical Division)
Extrapyramidal disorders in childhood
L. Angelini et al. editors

CHILDHOOD CHOREAS

SUSANNA ROLANDO, MAURIZIO DE NEGRI

Divisione e Cattedra di Neuropsichiatria Infantile

Istituto " Giannina Gaslini ". Università di Genova

INTRODUCTION

According to the classification of the Research Group on Extrapyramidal Disorders (21) "chorea is a state of excessive, spontaneous movements, irregularly timed, non repetitive, randomly distributed and abrupt in character. It may vary in severity from restlessness with mild intermittent exaggeration of gesture and expression, fidgeting movements of the hands, unstable dance-like gait to a continuous flow of disabling, violent movements".

While this disturbance is clearly recognizable in adults, simply by clinical observation, diagnosis in the infant and the very young child, whose motor activity is extremely lively, jerky and sudden, is more difficult.

The possibility of a " physiological chorea" or rather "pseudochorea" is accepted in infants, especially between the ages of two and five months, and is characterized by spontaneous rapid, twitching movements, increasing with excitement and apparently non purposive. Later on, in the preschool and school age range, some children retain a pattern of hyperkinesia closely resembling chorea that is not due to true pathology but to a maturational problem, gradually improving with growth. The postural instability is the main feature, while a normal ability to perform motor tasks is retained. Wallon (37) denominated this condition "subchoreic motor instability", Wolff and Hurwitz (38) used the term "choreiform syndrome". Frequently this motor pattern is associated with other signs of minimal cerebral dysfunction. Presumably in normal infants or in children with dysharmonic brain maturation, the regulatory action exerced by the association cortex on the motor cortex through the striatonigral system (1) is defective or delayed, and spontaneous motor activity has not yet acquired the purposiveness that makes the differentiation between voluntary and involuntary movements easy in adults. In childhood the diagnosis of chorea may therefore on occasion prove difficult. Laboratory examinations afford no definite help while electrophysiology can only add supportive information.

The EMG recordings in fact show a muscle activity very similar to voluntary contractions even though more fragmented and irregular (34). In Huntington chorea (H.C.) agonist and antagonist muscles are sometimes synchronously activated, but in most of childhood choreas (i.e. rheumatic as well as benign familial chorea) the spontaneous activity involves only the agonist muscles. According to Marsden (24) there is no characteristic pattern of EMG activity in chorea. The diagnosis of this disorder is therefore still essentially on clinical grounds.

Several biochemical pathways appear to be involved in chorea: a hyperactive nigrostriatal dopaminergic output, a defective striatal cholinergic and GABAergic activity have been demonstrated in H.C. Despite growing knowledge of the activity of various brain neurotransmitters and of the morphological changes in the basal ganglia, a common pathophysiological mechanism for all types of chorea has not yet been identified.

The clinical reponse to drugs is accordingly inconsistent. As well known, DOPA worsens H.C. (19), has no effect on chronic juvenile chorea (16), while it may be helpful in paroxysmal kinesigenic choreoathetosis (23). Such GABAergic compounds as sodium valproate fail to improve H.C. but relieve chorea caused by rheumatic infection (9, 26) Haloperidol has some efficacy on paroxysmal dystonic choreoathetosis but is detrimental in paroxysmal kinesigenic choreoathetosis (31). The efficacy of antiepileptic drugs in paroxysmal kinesigenic choreoathetosis is the only example of such therapeutic activity in extrapyramidal disorders.

Atrophy of the caudate nucleus has pointed to this structure as site of the primary process in this disorder. In H.C. neuronal degeneration in the neostriatum is associated with cellular dropout in cortical areas especially in the frontal cortex. On the other hand, in Sydenham disease or in lupus-associated chorea widespread inflammatory changes are prominent. Finally in other diseases, such as in paroxysmal choreoathetosis, pathological C N S changes are lacking.

Failure to identify a common biochemical or pathological process means that any classification of chorea in childhood is necessarily based upon the clinical features and traditional nosology. We will therefore consider the hereditary choreas and the choreas secondary to toxic, pharmacological and inflammatory causes in the light of the peculiarities of developmental age.(tab.1).

HEREDITARY CHOREAS

Huntington chorea in children

Huntington chorea (H.C.) is extremely infrequent in childhood. The prevalence of the disease in western countries is nearly 50 per 10^6. Cases with onset below the age of 20 account for 5 to 10% of the total number (5). Children usually have the rigid-hypokinetic form, and nearly always the affected parent is the father (7 times more often than the mother). This is probably due to a maternal (mitochondrial or X-chromosomal) protective factor (8) or a spermatic modifying gene (6). Early age at onset, presence of rigidity and paternal transmission are associated with a poorer prognosis (mean duration of illness in the juvenile rigid form is 11.0 + 5.1) (11).

We report as example a personal case: A.A. male, whose father, paternal grandmother and two aunts all had H.C., aged 5 at first observation, was reported to have developed normally until the age of 3. Gradually verbal function deteriorated and speech became poor and barely comprehensible. Progressive loss of initiative and interest led to withdrawal from peers, but the patient was still able to comunicate with his mother. At the age of 5 he was an expressionless, dysarthric boy, unable to dress or feed himself, walking a slow gait, without associated arm swinging movements. Neurological examination showed marked rigidity and pyramidal signs(Babinski sign and hyperreflexia), truncal titubation and broadbased gait; oculomotor apraxia and tremor, which are frequently associated with the akinetic rigid form of H.C. were not present in our case.

EEG showed slight slow irregularities

CT brain scan showed enlargement of the ventricular system with no cortical atrophy, suggesting caudate atrophy.

Familial benign chorea

Familial benign chorea or chronic juvenile chorea was first described by Haerer in 1966 (13). Since then nearly 100 cases have been reported (4) from several countries, including Italy (39).

The clinical features of all reported cases are fairly homogeneous. Onset is in the first decade; in a few cases the disease was already present in the first months of life. Involuntary movements are prevalent on the upper limbs and face. The lower limbs are less involved, although gait is clumsly with frequent falls, espe-

cially in the youngest children. Speech and intelligence are not affected but
school performance is impaired, due to writing and drawing difficulties. The disease is either stationary or improves with age.

A hereditary enzyme defect at dopaminergic pathway level is the supposed pathogenetic mechanism underlying this disorder.

In 20 of the 24 reported families, an autosomal pattern of transmission is evident. Penetrance is however incomplete (13) and this may probably explain the apparent horizontal distribution in some families.

The following personal case may exemplify the genetic pattern: A.A. is a seven
year old girl, reported " always " to have had motor problems, due to hyperkinesia, which disturbs gait, writing and drinking from a glass. At examination she
is an intelligent, cooperative girl, showing choreic movements of the limbs, trunk
and face and mild hypotonia. No pyramidal signs, ataxia or oculomotor defects are
present. Her stepsister, by the same father, clearly manifested the same symptoms
with a remitting course. Now at the age of 20, this half-sibling of our patient
shows minimal choreic movements of the upper limbs. The father refused to be examined, stating that he was "normal". The pattern of transmission of the disease in
our family is clearly dominant, either with low penetrance or low expressivity in
the father, even if a single sibship seems to be affected.

Paroxysmal Choreoathetosis

Attacks of choreic movements and dystonic posturing of the trunk and limbs, lasting minutes to hours, characterize this syndrome, first described by Mount and
Reback in 1940 (27).

Onset is in infancy or in the first years of life and the disorder is not associated with interictal neurological signs, shortened life span or tendency to
deterioration.

The attacks are frequently preceded by a prodromal sensation of tightness or
stiffness and are characterized by generalized choreic, ballistic and dystonic movements. To underline the prominence of the postural and tone change, Richards
proposed to call this syndrome " Paroxysmal Dystonic Choreoathetosis "(32).

Many different provocative factors are known, none of which is specific, except
alcohol. Caffeine, chocolate or tea are other possible trigger substances. Some
patients report an association with tiredness, fatigue or cold. Attacks never oc-

cur during sleep. Interictal as well as ictal EEG is normal.

Of the various drugs used, probably only the benzodiazepines have a definite, though short lived, therapeutic effect. Haloperidol and valproic acid have been claimed to have a beneficial effect by Przuntek and Monninger (31).

The pattern of transmission of the disease is clearly autosomal dominant in most of the reported families.

Paroxysmal Kinesigenic Choreoathetosis

The separation of this hereditary syndrome from paroxysmal non-kinesigenic choreoathetosis is not only due to the diversivity of precipitating factors but also to several other clinical characteristics that were stressed by Kertesz in 1967 (17) and then furtherly revised by Lance (22) and Goodenough (12).

Age of onset is somewhat later, usually during school age.

Attacks are provoked by a sudden movement after a period of rest; they are briefer than in P.D.C., lasting no more than 5 minutes, usually 20 to 30 seconds, and tend to recur many times a day. Frequently the abnormal movements are confined to one side of the body, or begin on one side and then rapidly spread to become bilateral.

There is always a good response to antiepileptic drugs, either phenobarbital, carbamazepine, valproate or phenytoin. Loong and Ong (23) reported a favorable effect of L-Dopa in one patient.

We recently observed a family with five affected members, a mother and four sons, in whom spontaneous remission occurred between the ages of 25 and 28 years. The symptoms started in all patients at the age of 11 to 13; the attacks were preceeded by a sensation of " insects crawling" on one limb, then violent, ballistic unilateral movements occurred and were followed by choreoathetosis lasting 1 to 5 minutes. The mother and the two older sons, aged 32 and 29, no longer have atta - cks. In the younger boys, aged 23 and 13, low dosage carbamazepine (200 mg daily) completely controlls the symptoms.

ACQUIRED CHOREAS

Rheumatic chorea

The incidence of Sydenham Chorea (S.C.) is decreasing, as well as other manifestations of rheumatic infection, but this disease is still the most common form of acute chorea in childhood, at least in our country.

In the last ten years 13 patients have been admitted to our hospital for subacute or acute chorea associated with behavioural disturbances, anxiety, listlesness. S.C. was diagnosed on the basis of the clinical and laboratory examinations and follow-up.

Our data are similar to those published in the literature (28). Age at onset was 6 to 14 years (median age 10.4 yrs). Male to female ratio was 1:3. Chorea was predominant unilaterally in 4 cases and generalized in 9. In all cases the past history was suggestive of streptococcal infection either angina (11 case) or nodosus erythema (2 case)or scarlet fever (1 case). Biological tests always showed an increased erythrocyte sedimentation rate, even if slight, and a high anti-O-streptolysin title (250 to 3000 U/1). More inconstantely an increase of alpha-2-globulins or C protein or a positivite throat culture has been found. Cardiac involvement was not demonstrate in spite of extensive and periodically repeated investigations (EKG, Xray, Echocardiography). This contrasts with previously reported data (2,28) and either reflects the smallness of our sample or the improvement in treatment in the last decades in terms of timeliness and prolonged maintenance of antibiotic prophylaxis.

The close relationship between S.C. and rheumatic fever was recognized in the late XIX century and is now so well established that in cases without evidence of serological positivity for group A streptococcal infections, other possible causes of acute chorea should be more likely considered.

Although the pathogenesis of S.C. is still unknown, the discovery in the blood of IgG antibodies against neuronal cytoplasmic antigens of the caudate and subthalamic nuclei is convincing evidence of an immunological mechanism (15). This finding supports the hypothesis of a cross-reaction between antistreptococcal antibodies and basal ganglia antigens.

From a pathological point of view, no specific morphological changes have been found in the few post mortem examinations. Diffuse neuronal degenerative changes are present in the basal ganglia as well as in the cerebral and cerebellar cortex. Perivascular inflammatory infiltrates and necrotizing arteritis are also frequently observed. The prevalence of pathological changes in the caudate and putamen nuclei is frequently but not always reported. Nevertheless the central role of the striatus in the pathogenesis of S.C. is supported by the symptomatological similarity to H.C. and the response to drugs.

Results of therapeutic trials suggest hyperactivity of dopaminergic system. In fact, reserpine, which reduces the dopamine-content in the striatus and chloropromazine and haloperidol, which have central dopamine receptor blocking activity, considerably reduce choreic movements in S.C., as in H.C. (19).Further, the therapeutic effects of drugs like valproate, presumably reflect an abnormality of the GABAergic pathway also (9,26).

Treatment is both causal and symptomatic. We chose to prolong antibiotic therapy, preferably with benzathine-penicillin, for at least three years. Symptomatic treatment includes a variety of tranquilizers (frequently used are benzodiazepines), antidopaminergic agents such as haloperidol or GABAergic drugs, particularly valproate.

Chorea in Systemic Lupus Erythematosus

Systemic Lupus Erythematosus (S.L.E.) may be responsible for various neurological symptoms such as seizures, psychosis, focal neurological deficits. Chorea is a rare manifestation of S.L.E. and nearly always affects children or young adults. Herd and al. (14) reviewed 36 published cases. The age at onset was 16 years or less in 53% of patients and under 20 years in 64%. In 11 patients chorea was the presenting symptom.

The differential diagnosis from S.C. may be difficult: the clinical symptoms, age at onset, female prevalence, mean duration, are similar in both diseases and a misdiagnosis of S.C. is nearly the rule when involuntary movements precede other manifestations of S.L.E.
The chorea is not related to the stage or the severity of the underlying disease or to other neurological or visceral symptoms.

A vascular disturbance, caused by occlusion of the small vessels of the basal ganglia is the presumed pathological substrate (17). Alternatively an autoimmune mechanism, due to cytotoxic antibodies reacting with neuronal antigens, as S.C., has been proposed (3).

Therapy is directed essentially to the primary disease since involuntary movements as a rule recede as the illness improves, making symptomatic treatment with haloperidol unnecessary except in the most severe cases and for a limited period.

Drug-induced and toxic chorea

An extensive list of drugs that may cause chorea is reported by Padberg and

Bruyn (30).

Apart from the well known dyskinesia caused by neuroleptic and dopaminergic drugs, several other substances have on rare occasions been responsible for the onset of choreic movements.

The possible harmfulness of oral contraceptive must be borne in mind by the pediatric neurologist following young patients who suffered from rheumatic chorea. Most of the reported cases in fact are adolescent girls with a prior history of S.C.

Central nervous system stimulants, d-amphetamine, methylphenidate and pemoline, are used in children with minimal brain dysfunction (" attention deficit"). At toxic doses these drugs may cause an acute chorea. A chronic chorea is also possible at therapeutic dosage, especially in children with previous signs of encephalopathy. The mechanism is probably a facilitating effect on the striatal dopamine receptors.

Other possible causes of chorea are antiepileptic drugs, especially phenytoin, carbamazepine and phenobarbital. A toxic blood level is not always present, but in most cases chronic high-dose polytherapy is the supposed cause. Particularly prone to develop involuntary movements are children with underlying cerebral lesions. A possible common mechanism for the action of these antiepileptic drugs on the serotonergic and dopaminergic striatal activity has been suggested (20).

Carbon monoxide intoxication commonly causes parkinsonism in adults; a delayed and transient chorea has rarely been reported. We observed an acute, extremely violent, choreic syndrome in a 13 year old boy who, four days before, had been found unconscious following accidental CO intoxication. Conscioussness was soon restored and he was perfectly well for four days, till the onset of the abnormal movements. Within a week, on phenotyazine therapy, the chorea completely disappeared. Similar cases have been reported by Schwartz (35) and Davous (7).

CHOREOATHETOSIS PRECEDING DYSTONIA

Involuntary movements are often observed in inherited metabolic diseases with widespread cerebral involvement. In some cases chorea or choreoathethosis may be the presenting and main symptom, as for example in ataxia teleangectasia, gradually giving place to, or being overshadowed by other signs of central nervous system impairment. It is not uncommon to see a modification of dyskinetic movements in the course of progressive childhood diseases, and when this happens a shift from a hyperkinetic to a hypokinetic-rigid form is likely. As we are not dealing with progressive metabolic disorders, which will be discussed elsewhere in this volume, we will report and discuss four cases of " idiopathic ", non progressive, extra-pyramidal syndromes, in which a modification of the involuntary movement pattern has been observed and videotaped over the course of years.

Case 1 (B W) is a 7 year old boy followed by us since the age of four (33). On attainment of upright posture and locomotion, rapid irregular involuntary move-ments of the lower limbs were evident, giving way to a bizarre dancing gait. Al-though unable to stand still or to walk on a straight line, he never lost his balance. Gradually this choreic syndrome receded and ceased after the age of four, but, at this time, dystonic spasms of the lower limbs, (flexion-inversion of one or both feet) appeared. They were observed only in the late afternoon and evening and low-dosage L-dopa therapy completely inhibited them. Now, at the age of seven, this boy appears to be affected by a fluctuating dystonia similar to the condi-tion reported by Segawa (8, 36).

Case 2 (B M) is a mentally subnormal 23 year old girl, followed since the age of 14. She suffers from marked rigidity associated with hypokinesia and dystonic limbs posturing. The mother reported that in infancy and early childhood she was very " active" though a mental deficit was already evident and did not worsen with age. During the 9 year follow up no deterioration occurred.

Case 3 and 4 (B Ba and B Br) twins, are the sisters of case 2 and first came to our attention at age 7 months. They have always been retarded, like the older sister, and since the first years of life have presented generalized choreo-athe-totic movements. Now, at age 9 years, they are becoming less and less choreic and dystonic posturing, especially of the lower limbs, is appearing. We believe that the three girls have the same familial extrapyramidal syndrome, whose clini-cal signs are changing with age, without evidence of true deterioration.

DISCUSSION

Chorea has been observed in a variety of syndromes, may be part of the signs and simptoms of metabolic and degenerative disorders, or may be provoked by diffe-rent insults. It is therefore an aspecific sign frequently observed in childhood and adolescence; indeed children seem to be more susceptible than adults to deve-lop choreic symptoms.

This is the case with the hyperkinesia induced by antiepileptic drugs, especially hydantoin and carbamazepine. While in adults abnormal movements appear at toxic blood levels, this is not always so in children.

Chorea gravidarum and chorea associated with oral contraceptive drugs usually affect very young women. The median age of reported cases is lower than the median childbearing age. Patients of 20 or less account for 40% in the Nausieda revision of estro-progestinic induced chorea and only two patients (0.8%) were over 25 (29).

As seen previously, diseases which occur in both adults and children, like rheumatic fever and SLE, are rarely responsible for a choreic syndrome after childhood.

Primary idiopathic hereditary disorders in many cases affect children and adolescents and improve or are completely overcome with age. This is so in benign familial chorea and paroxysmal kinesigenic choreoathetosis.

Chorea may be the presenting and main symptom in more complex idiopathic or metabolic disorders, gradually giving way to signs of involvement of other systems.

Extrapyramidal syndromes of childhood may show a progressive modification from a hyperkinetic, choreic or choreoathetosic pattern of movement, to a hypokinetic-rigid or dystonic syndrome.

Taking these examples and considerations together we would say that chorea is a facilitated symptom in the first years of life. This is especially true of the familial benign syndromes or those caused by toxic and pharmacological agents in which a biochemical derangement is presumable. Degenerative disorders, due to neuronal loss such as H.C. or Choreaocantocytosis do not have this age prevalence.

Biochemical studies on brain neurotransmitters (25) disclosed a different enzymatic activity at different ages. The dopa-synthetizing enzyme tyroxine hydroxylase (TH) has high values in the caudate, putamen and nucleus accumbens of children and decreases very sharply till the age of 20 yrs and more slowly afterwards. The same, though to a lesser degree, happens with glutamate decarboxylase (GAD) and choline acetyltransferase (CAT).

Dopaminergic nerve axons of the caudate and putamen arise from cell bodies in the substantia nigra. The reduction in the number of cells of the substantia nigra is not by itself sufficient to explain the dramatic dropout of TH between the ages of 5 and 25 years.

It appears therefore that decreased enzymatic activity in this period is not only due to cell loss but chiefly to a still unknown metabolic mechanism.

The decrease of dopaminergic function with age could be correlated to the improvement of familial choreic syndromes, the rarity of inflammatory, toxic and pharmacological choreas in adults and the modification of complex encephalopathies from an hyperkinetic toward a rigid-hypokinetic extrapyramidal symptomatology.

More has to be learned about pathological and biochemical changes in extrapyramidal movement disorders and research is greatly improving our knowledges.

From a clinician's point of view it is important to stress the need of more longitudinal studies and of an adequate follow up of single cases as extrapyramidal disorders in children have a dynamic and age-correlate expressivity.

TABLE 1

HEREDITARY CHOREAS

Huntington Chorea

Benign Familial Chorea

Paroxysmal Chorea or Choreoathetosis

              non Kinesigenic (dystonic)

              Kinesigenic

Chorea in inherited metabolic diseases

ACQUIRED CHOREAS

Lesional

              Perinatal Encephalopathies

              Trauma

              Vascular lesions

Inflammatory

              Rheumatic Chorea

              Chorea in S.L.E.

Toxic

              drugs

              CO

REFERENCES

1. Allen GI, Tzukahara N(1974) Physiol Rev 54:957-1006

2. Aron A, Freeman J, Carter S(1965) Am J Med 28:83-95

3. Atkins CJ, London JJ, Quismorio FP, Frion GJ (1972) Ann Intern Med 76:65-72

4. Bruyn GW, Mirianthopoulos NC (1986) In: Vinken PJ, Bruyn GW, Klawans HL(eds) Handbook of Clinical Neurology. Elsevier, Amsterdam, pp 335-348

5. Bruyn GW, Went LN (1986) In: Vinken PJ, Bruyn GW, Klawans HL (eds) Handbook of Clinical Neurology. Elsevier, Amsterdam, pp 267-313

6. Bundey S (1985) Genetics and Neurology.Churchill Livingstone, Edinburgh, pp 95-101

7. Davous P, Rondot P, Marion MH, Queguen B (1986) J Neurol Neurosurg Psychiatr 49:206-208

8. Deonna T (1986) Neuropediatrics 17:75-80

9. Dhanaray M, Radhaktishan AR (1985) Neurology 35:114-115

10. Farrer CA, Conneally PM (1985) Am J Hum Genet 37: 350-357

11. Farrer CA, Conneally PM (1987) Arch Neurol 44: 109-113

12. Goodenough DJ, Fariello RG, Annis BL, Chun RWM (1978) Arch Neurol 35:827-831

13. Haerer AF, Currier RD, Jackson JF (1966) Neurology: 307

14. Herd JK, Medhi M, Uzendoski DM, Saldivar VA (1978) Pediatrics 61:308-315

15. Husby G, Van De Rijn I, Zabriskie JB (1976) J Exp Med 144: 1094-1110

16. Ito T, Suzuki H, Yamada M (1982) Brain Nerve 34: 775-780

17. Johnson RT, Richardson EP (1968) Medicine 47: 337-369

18. Kertèsz A (1967) Neurology 17:680-690

19. Klawans HL, Weiner WJ (1981) Textbook of Clinical Neuropharmacology. Raven Press, New York, pp 49-67

20. Krishnamoorthy KS, Zalneraitis EL, Young RSK, Bernard PG (9183) Pediatrics 72: 831-834

21. Lakke PWF, Barbeau A, Duvoisin RC, Gerstenbrand K, Marsden CD, Stern G (1981) J Neurol Sci 51:311-327

22. Lance JW (1977) Ann Neurol 2: 285-293

23. Long SC, Ong YY (1973) J Neurol Neurosurg Psychiatr 36: 921-924

24. Marsden CD, Obeso JA, Rothwell JC (1983) In : Desmedt JE (ed) Motor Control Mechanisms in Health and Disease. Raven Press, New York, pp 865-881

25. Mc Geer PL, Mc Geer EG, Suzuki JS(1977) Arch Neurol 34: 33-35

26. Mc Lachlan RS (1981) Br Med J 283: 274-275

27. Mount LA, Reback S (1940) Arch Neurol 44: 841- 846

28. Nausieda PA, Grossman BJ, Koller WC (1980) Neurology 30: 331-334

29. Nausieda PA, Koller WC, Weiner WJ, Klawans HL (1980) Neurology 30: 1131-1132

30. Padberg GW, Bruyn GW (1986) In: Vinken PJ, Bruyn GW, Klawans HL (eds) Handbook of Clinical Neurology . Elsevier, Amsterdam, pp 549-564

31. Przuntek H, Monninger P (1983) J Neurol 230: 163-169

32. Richards RN, Barnett HJM (1968) Neurology 18: 461-499

33. Rolando S, Rasmini P Revue Neurol (in press)

34. Rondot P (1983) Neuropediatrics 14: 59-65

35. Schwartz A, Hennerici M, Wegener OH (1985) Neurology 35: 98-99

36. Segawa M, Hosaka A, Miygawa F, Nomura Y, Imai H (1976) Adv Neurol 14: 215-233

37. Wallon H (1925) L'enfant turbulent. Alcan, Paris

38. Wolff PH, Hurwitz I (1966) Dev Med Child Neurol 8: 160-165

39. Zambrino CA, La Buonora I, Lanzi G, Burgio FR (1984) G Neuropsichiatr Età Evol 4: 81-87.

© 1987 Elsevier Science Publishers B.V. (Biomedical Division)
Extrapyramidal disorders in childhood
L. Angelini et al. editors

TICS AND GILLES DE LA TOURETTE SYNDROME

UMBERTO BALOTTIN, CARLO ALBERTO ZAMBRINO, GIOVANNI LANZI

Child Neuropsychiatry Division, Fondazione Mondino, University of Pavia, Via
Palestro 3, 27100 Pavia

In 1885, there appeared an article in the journal "Archives de Neurologie",
written by George Gilles de la Tourette entitled:" Etude sur une affection
nerveuse caractérisée par l'incoordination motrice accompagnée de echolalie e
de coprolalie" (19). In it, this student of Charcot, described a "bizzarre"
pathology characterized by involuntary movements and multiple tics, accompanied
by unrestrained vocalizations, often obscene in nature.

Over a century has passed since the original description, and although the
clinical characteristics were well noted, many problems concerning GTS remain
as yet unsolved. This syndrome elicited a common interest for those phenomena
which bordered between neurology and psychiatry, and for which the interactions
among the "organic" and "functional" characteristics still remain difficult to
comprehend.

Problems also arise in defining the nosographic and physiopathogenetic
correlations between GTS and other tic manifestations, in particular, simple
tics.

Based upon numerous observations (42, 43) which demonstrate the efficacy of
haloperidol in controlling the tics of GTS, it is possible to hypothesize a
specific effect of the drug in relation to its activity at the level of monoaminergic receptors. On the one hand, this data is indicative of a possible
neurochemical alteration involving diffuse regulatory systems, while on the
other hand, it gives us little information regarding the possible functional
circuits eventually involved in the genesis of the tics. This is also in
relation to the fact that this disturbance comprehends distinct
psychopatologic aspects, but at the same time, has an indisputable pathogenetic basis of organic origin.

Besides the clinical standpoint, simple and complex tics appear distinct in
their electrophysiologic characteristics. Simple tics, are in fact connotated
by arythmic, brief episodes which are synchronous or slightly asynchronous
with agonist-antagonist muscles.

Complex tics show a greater variability in electrophysiologic data, where contrarily, the activation and contemporaneous inhibition of agonist-antagonist may allow the presence of a normal ballistic movement.

Therefore, observations may include aspects of different, albeit pathologic, movements as expression, from time to time, of a possible defect in the control of reciprocal innervation, or of the finalization and intentionality of the movement itself, which nonetheless conserves characteristics of normality during its phases.

The possible relationships between the electrical activity registered at the scalp level and electromyographic potentials were studied in the Tourette Syndrome by Obeso and coll. (37). The demonstration of the absence of a premovement negative potential ("bereitschaftpotential") immediately before the onset of motor tics, indicates that the tics are functionally distinct from voluntary movement, since they are characterized by automaticity, are involuntary, and are not under the control of conscious mental processes.

Thus, a possible correlation exists between motor tics and other pathologic manifestations of Known subcortical origin, in particular, at the level of the basal nuclei. Clinical observations then demonstrated that tic manifestations also appeared during the course of post-encephalitic Parkinson's disease and tardive dyskinesia (12, 25). The analysis of semeiological characteristics of tics has shown similarities with other extrapyramidal pathologies: the "repetition" and "iteration", the involvement of rythmic and mimical-emotive movements, constitute further proof of a possible relationship between the diverse pathologies.

It is therefore correct, when referring to motor tics, to speak of spontaneous activation of acquired motor sequences, that is, elementary components of the more complex phase of movement. It is also Known that the basal nuclei have the role of controlling the activation and simultaneous inhibition of the agonist and antagonist muscle groups, in addition to the planning of how and when the motor activity arises, through the nigrostriatal and strio-pallidal circuits.

The conceptual definition of involuntariness, regarding the tic syndromes, includes evident limitations. The concurrence of subjectively experienced pregestual compulsions, consequently released through anxiety, and the ability to control the frequency of his tics for a certain period of time (nontheless successively worsened) are indications that the emotional aspects of movement and the expression of aggressive emotions using the somatomotor system, play an important role.

On the other hand it has not been possible to obtain experimental models of GTS, nor has a histopathological investigation given convincing results (14); this gives further support to the hypothesis which emphasizes the important correlations between emotions and learning-conditioning phenomena in the genesis of tic syndromes. Therefore, according to certain authors, it is more feasible that a possible neurochemical dysfunction is not attributable to the nigrostriatal circuits, but to the mesocortical components which control emotions and which are able to elicit adaptive and aggressive behaviors.

The study of the phenomena associated with motor tics in GTS supports the hypothesis of a probable multisystemic deficit.

Studies using PET (7) have observed an inverse correlation between the severity of vocal tics and glucose metabolism at the level of the language cortex. The velocity of utilization of glucose had been demonstrated to be about 15% less in the frontal, insular, cingular, and inferior striatal body regions. This hypofunction at cortical levels and of striatal regions seems to be a compensatory pre-synaptic mechanism of hypersensitive, post-synaptic dopaminergic receptors.

According to other authors, the coprolalia of GTS could be considered a chance phenomenon, due to the greater or lesser ease with which the combination of syllables or phonetics of a certain language may lead to assonances that recall vulgar terms. This could explain the different frequence of occurrence of coprolalia according to the mother tongue.

Other phenomena, such as ecolalia, ecoprassia and mental coprolalia (which has a more evident psychopathologic component), remain as yet difficult to explain.

GTS also commonly shares with other extrapyramidal pathologies, its etiology as a neurovegetative dysfunction. This becomes manifest as a modification in the normal equilibrium between the sympathetic and parsympathetic systems (41). Thus, hypothetically, it may be considered as a defect and/or dysfunction of the circuits connecting the basal ganglia, hypothalamus and the mesodiencephalic and pontomedullary structures.

Based upon the above information, it would surely be arbitrary to formulate any conclusive statements.

Simple and complex tics may be defined as a disturbance in the finalization of a movement which involves emotional components of the subject, and thus, the mesolimbic projections. GTS, instead, seems to be characterized by a multisystemic involvement of different functional circuits. The heterogeneity of symptoms, the evolution of the syndrome, and the relationships with tic manifestations, could all be due to a variability of the phenotypes which comprehend distinct genotypes found in different physiopathological anomalies.

We will now present, in more detail, the epidemiology, the genetics, and the studies of neurochemistry and psychodynamics relative to GTS.

EPIDEMIOLOGY/GENETICS

The problems involved in achieving a better understanding of GTS are seen when attempting to interpret epidemiological data. Discordance between the diverse results seems to be a great deal. Salami (40) reports one case in every 5,300 children, with an incidence of 1.9: 10,000. Asher (1) reports an incidence rate of 0.7: 10,000.

The Tourette Syndrome Association and the DSM-III estimate the incidence of GTS to be 1-5 per 10,000.

Cohen reports a prevalence of 1: 2,000 in Conneticut, while Burd (4) reports 5.2: 10,000 in North Dakota in a population of 140,580 school age children.

These numbers refer to the complete clinical expression of the syndrome, and only the most recent studies used diagnostic criteria standardized by DSM-III, which partially explains the difference in results. It is certain that there is a prevalence in the male sex, with variabilities according to the different authors, between 3:1 and 9.3:1.

The genetic approach has been recently developed. Familial cases of GTS have shown an aggregation of the full syndrome with vocal and motor multiple tics (23, 24, 36). It remains to be seen if these actually represent a different spectrum of the same disorder; in this case, the prevalence of a predisposition for GTS could be approximately equal to 1: 200 or 1: 300.

Clinical studies using monozigotic twins have demonstrated high concordance in the prevalence, nontheless, of a highly variable symptomatology such that one may think of a possible influence from external factors (ie., psychopathologic or pre-/post-natal events) upon gene expression.

Thus, our further considerations can only refer to the numerous points of this aspect as yet unresolved. It is not possible to define a pattern of Mendelian transmission of GTS, although one has been hypothesized, but not confirmed, regarding an autosomal dominant mode of inheritance. The genetic penetrance is surely not complete, and it is probable that a fair amount of cases, especially during childhood, are not correctly diagnosed. The use of recombinant DNA techniques for linkage mapping have not, to the present time, supplied convincing results, even if they open interesting prospectives for the future. This also applies to the studies pertaining to the identification of possible antigenic or enzymatic markers (11).

NEUROCHEMICAL APPROACH

The efficacy of haloperidol in controlling the tics of GTS appears to be a sufficiently confirmed result, even though, as Marsden (33) reports, both the physiopathologic and neurochemical mechanisms involved in GTS are not known. One must also consider that this efficacy is not generalized to all, since it is possible to identify subjects which do not respond to the drug, and above all, admit that the drug has never, or almost never, had absolute therapeutic efficacy. It can give obvious improvement, but not complete resolution of the disturbance; the latter, instead, may be seen in certain extrapyramidal diseases better defined as dystonia Parkinsonims syndrome. Also, the value of this drug for its placebo effect should not be underestimated.

The therapeutic benefits from haloperidol are nonetheless superior to those of other drug categories, such as the phenothiazines; this hypothesizes a specific effect for the drug. In addition, the administration of methyl-phenidate and dextroamphetamine (13), dopaminergic antagonists, induce a worsening in the frequency of motor tics. Thus, it seems feasible to hypothesize that the genesis of motor tics is due to a possible functional pre valence of monoaminergic systems, in particular, to a hypersensitivity of the dopaminergic receptor (44, 46). In favor of this hypothesis is the observation of low basal levels of HVA in the liquor of patients with GTS, which indicates a feed-back inhibition upon dopaminergic turnover. In fact, following a postsynaptic receptor blockage with haloperidol, there is a successive increase in liquor levels of HVA (9).

For other dopaminergic antagonist drugs, a therapeutic efficacy has also been observed for pimozide and fluphenazine, with analogous actions to haloperidol upon postsynaptic receptors, in the treatment of GTS. Also, tetrabenazine (already useful for the therapy of other hyperkinetic disorders such as Huntington's disease, tardive dyskinesia, and dystonia) has the advantage over haloperidol of having less side effects. In this sense, the drug's effect seems to be correlated not as much to the receptor blockade, as to a pre-synaptic action of monoaminergic depletion (similarly to alfa-methyl-para-tyrosine and reserpine) by enzymatic inhibition of its synthesis (22).

Neurochemical comparisons and therapeutic trials also support the possible involvement of other neurotransmitters. Therefore, considering the hypothesis of an altered function of the dopaminergic systems at the basal ganglia level, one must theoretically take into consideration the possibility of an altered equilibrium between dopaminergic and cholinergic circuits; the relative predominance of the former may be attributable to a relative cholinergic hypofunction (as in Huntington's disease). The demonstration of a preponderant parasympathetic activity in GTS appears to confirm this theory. An increase in the concentration of acetycholine, associated with a decrease in the activity of the specific and non-specific serum acetylcholinesterase, and an elevated concentration of intracellular choline, has been reported by various authors. Also, the modifications of cardiac activity, reported by Schelkunov and others, in GTS, are indications of an altered cholinergic/dopaminergic equilibrium, not only at the striatal level, but also at the ponto-medullary level (41).

Based upon this hypothesis, various studies have been performed in order to evaluate the efficacy of cholinergic drugs in GTS (2, 38, 45), which nevertheless, have not given unanimous results. The i.v. administration of physostigmine (a cholinesterase inhibitor) in six patients with GTS, resulted in a decreased frequency of motor tics for six hours, and the effect was unaltered by successive administration of propantheline (an antagonist to the cholinergic activity of physostigmine). The use of lecithin and of choline chlorhydrate gave contradictory results (38). In other experiments, following

the administration of scopolamine (a cholinergic receptor blocker), there was
a decrease in the frequency of motor tics, while use of physostigmine worsened
the frequency of tics. Contrarily, the effect was exactly the opposite upon
verbal tics, which led the Authors to formulate a hypothetical cholinergic
genesis of verbal tics, different from motor tics (45). The apparently positive
results obtained with the administration of serotonin precursors, such as 5-HTP
in combination with carbidopa, suggest that serotoninergic circuits may be
involved in GTS (46). These data have not as yet receive further support; in
fact, there are reports of negative effects following the administration of
serotonin precursors.

Certain researchers postulate that, based upon observations obtained from
animal models, serotoninergic circuits may be involved in the genesis of simple
tics, which are functionally distinct from complex tics interpreted by
"dopaminergic models" (analogously to the stereotypical mannerisms induced by
administration of amphetamino derivatives).

The favorable therapeutic effect of clonidine (10, 30) in some patients with
GTS has called attention to the possible participation of central noradrenergic
systems, preferentially mediated by α2-adrenergic presynaptic receptor sites.

An interesting observation was made in subjects with no response to
haloperidol, but therapeutically sensitive to clonidine (6). A link between the
two substances could be explained on the basis of a transynaptic influence by
the liberation of other neurotransmitters at the striatal level, mediated by
the activation of presynaptic receptors which do not depend upon cyclic AMP.

As yet, data relative to the efficacy of drug action upon GABA systems has
not been confirmed, although positive effects have been observed using N-dipro-
pylacetic acid.

The role of other neurotransmitters with known complex interactions in the
basal ganglia, and which participate in the genesis of other extrapyramidal
pathologies, still remains to be defined.

PSYCHOPATHOLOGICAL APPROACH

While underlining the interest in the neurobiological approach, it also
seems necessary to attentively consider the psychopathological approach to tics
and to the Gilles de la Tourette Syndrome.

It would seem limitative, to attribute the mental dysfunction to a conceptual dualism between the psychogenetic and organogenetic versions, without considering how the somatic expression (through the disorganization of biological systems) could construct, especially in childhood, the means to manifest the discomfort tied to the conflictual situation (27). In fact, the organogenetic hypotheses for tic manifestations find support primarily in the efficacy of neuroleptic treatments, nonetheless incomplete and not always continuous. Recalling examples of the relatively dubious and contradictory neurophysiological results, it would seem pretentious to initially eliminate any psychoanalytic psychopathological approach which nevertheless reports therapeutic efficacy (29).

One must remember, among many examples, the case description of child A., treated with complete success by C. Chiland, whose clinical course was followed until adulthood, or also, the case of little Abdelaziz described by Lebovici and coll. in a recent study. Similarly, in our clinic and ambulatory setting, we have had occasion to observe several times how a global intervention, addressed above all to the object-relation aspect, is able to determine net and durable improvements, even in grave cases of Tourette Syndrome.

Already, in the past, both tics and the Tourette Syndrome were considered simple expressions of madness or as pertaining to a syndrome which evolved towards alienation and dementia. Nonetheless, this type of evolution was never confirmed. Repeated presentations in journals of the organistic viewpoint, show cases of Tourette Syndrome which in adolescence evolved in psychoses (6).

This revised relationship between the more serious stages of psychopathology and the Tourette Syndrome, can be briefly reviewed by reading the description made by authors such as Elridge and Shapiro (15): they describe how certain behavioral characteristics, of their patients studied, gave information as to how they have common or similar originswith those which limit upon psychosis.

In such subjects, Eldridge describes exhibitionist behaviors in the family or public settings, frequent impulses to touch their mother's breasts, or to touch their own genitals in certain situations, etc.

Other authors, such as Bruun (5), describe in adult patients the grave incapacity to establish lasting relationships with a partner, vagabonding, suicidal tendencies, and repeated admissions to psychiatric hospitals. All these characteristics which have been described and easily observed many times before in clinical practice, are considered by authors with a monolateral vision of the syndrome, as pure consequences of the neurochemical disturbance.

On the other hand, our point of view considers these characteristics to be part of a complex psychopathological syndrome which expresses itself through movements, neurochemical alteration, and purely psychiatric symptomatology.

We shall now briefly describe the personality of a child with tics and of a child with tic disease.

We can distinguish, in accordance with Rouart (39), two different types of personalities. The first group comprehends children with tics which are characterized by good scholastic and socio-familial adjustment, and by the fact that the tic constitutes the only problematic element for the child, even if these children are anxious and infantile for their age.

The second group comprehends unstable, turbulent, hyperkinetic children. Margaret Mahler underlined that often, there is a continuity from the first to the second stage of childhood, in that the child whom at first was restless, always moving vivacious and uncontrollable, tends later on, in certain cases, to evolve into a child with tics.

Common characteristics of a child with tics include the ambivalence which occurs according to the obedient-rebellious personality, and the delayed developmentx of affect and infantilism, which Meige and Feindel (34) already described in their fundamental study as: "younger or older children with tics, present with a mental age inferior to that which is present in reality". It is also of note that a child which expresses a tic, also expresses an aggression towards his parents, which becomes masochistic the moment at which it evocates criticism and reproof from the adults. It is clear, that if these aspects of children with tics seem a bit contradictory and polymorphous, there is, nonetheless, general agreement as to the importance of repressed aggressive tendencies.

Colette Chiland, in a recent study (1983, 8) underlines that these patients differ from each other because their cases are on the borderline between different personality organizations and familial configuration. Nevertheless, there is an element common to all: a series of circumstances which cause the subject great difficulty when trying to handle his internal processes of hate.

In regards to the family of a child with tics it must be underlined that there is a certain frequency of previous psychiatric disorders among the parents, in particular, of obsessive neuroses.

The parental behavior towards their children is characterized by a tense and perfectionistic familial atmosphere in which quarrels and disputes are frequent. There is also a marked tendency to impose restrictions upon muscular movements, and not respect the child's bodily autonomy, with frequent physical interventions upon the child to help him or stop him. M. Mahler (32) retains that the maternal attitude is characterized by a mixture of anxiety, and rigidity.

This could explain why these children remain in an infantile emotional state. Also notable, in brief, are the typical familial reactions to the appearance of a tic.

The tics elicit familial disapproval with the tendency to prohibit and stop them, faced with the child's "bad behavior". These reactions give rise to feelings of intense guilt in the child. There is also the possibility that the tic elicits heated quarrels between members of the family which the child observes as an ambivalent spectator to a drama he himself has caused. Thus, he has no other choice, but to increase the persistence of his symptoms so that the tics become for the family, as some mothers note, a sort of "obsession".

It is evident that the tic often appears in the age when the Oedipal complex normally resolves, and thus permits the evolution towards latency. But, as is already clear, the conflicts and aggressiveness are the essential bases of the disturbance upon which these children lend support at stages more primitive to the development of affect, stages which are undoubtedly of the pre-Oedipal or pre-genital type.

All the authors who studied tics, from Janet and Charcot to Meige and Feindel, and still others, have always insisted upon the relationship between tics and obsessions. Despite the obsessive characteristics present in parents, it is also frequently observed that children with isolated tics have hidden, but distinct elements of an obsessive neurosis. In order to avoid lengthy clinical examples, we could briefly state that the tic in a child could be the motor equivalent of obsessions, of which the tic represents the prodrome.

The pathogenesis of the disturbance is classified in two groups, according to the authors who have studied it. Those such as Meige and Feindel consider tics as essentially cortical phenomena, whose genesis and maintenance depends upon the mental status of the subject. Others, on the other hand, insist upon the neurological aspects of tics, post-encephalitic tics, and upon the relationship between tics and extrapyramidal neurological phenomena.

At this point, the studies by Levy and Pacella (28) are noteworthy. They give great importance to the influence of restricted movements as possible initiators of a regression towards lower levels of psychophysiological integration. These authors underline the fact that observations of real tics occur in horses, and that certain movements of the horse's head, immobilized in his stall, are very similar to the tics observed in children.

On the other hand, it should be remembered that Thesi Bergmann, has shown that in occasions of prolonged restraint for bone fractures in children, no development of tics was observed.

Considering these modalities, so opposite in their approach to this problem, we believe that, in ultimate analysis, the classification proposed by Margaret Mahler (32), even if not completely accepted by successive authors, represents a mode of integrating the two viewpoints (organistic and psychodynamic) and accounts for the clinical and psychopathological polymorphism. She underlines in many works how the tics specific for GTS, represent organic neuroses whose tic symptom does not symbolize a conflict, but the direct physiological expression of a certain emotional background. She also notes that these children are anxious, depressed, inhibited and passive, all characteristics which describe essential depression, according to the French psychosomatic school of thought. In addition, the author states a statistical prevalence in males, whose neuromuscular apparatus is the elective site of psychological investement of aggression. Thus, for Mahler, the tic disease corresponds to a difficulty in integrating the psychomotor system under the control of the self. This is due to a particular modality of mental function which we may define as psychosomatic, but is also due to a true neuroorganic predisposition to manifest motor disturbances of this type.

Mahler also makes a distinction between tic disease or GTS, and temporary tics or tics symptomatic of a psychoneurosis (conversion hysteria and obsessive neurosis) or of a psychosis. This latter interpretation is already present in the case description given by Freud and Breuer of Emmy von N., (18) in whom the tics were seen as compromised solutions, through the conversion mechanism, of a conflict between representation and the tendency to suppress it.

In this manner, Ferenczi (16) affirmed that there was a close correlation between tics and narcissistic psychoneurosis.

In conclusion, putting aside the neuroorganic aspects which we have already considered at length, which represent the somatic basis of the disturbance, and probably, also the predispositional component, we have tried to delineate some of the major tendencies of the psychodynamic approach to this problem.

It remains to be seen if this is a unique pathology which borders between a transfert neurosis, an actual neurosis or psychosomatic illness, a narcissistic neurosis or psychosis, or if this is a syndrome of diverse clinical aspects with different underlying psychopathologic mechanisms.

In any case, despite the presence of an organic predisposition, which comprehends a pathological motor manifestation as the symptom of a specific psychopathologic syndrome, it still remains difficult to integrate the two different approaches (neurological and psychodynamic) into a borderline pathology, such as tics and GTS, which is generally resistant to the therapeutic trials presently available.

REFERENCES

1. Asher E (1948) Amer J Psychiat 105:267-275

2. Barbeau A (1980) N Engl J Med 302:1310-1311

3. Baron M, Shapiro A et al (1981) Am J Hum Genet 33: 767-775

4. Burd L, Kerbeshian J, Wikenheiser M, Fisher W (1986) J Am Acad Child Psychiatry 25, 4:552-553

5. Bruun RD (1984) J Am Acad Child Psychiatry 23, 2:126-133

6. Caine RD (1985) Arch Neurol 42:393-397

7. Chase TN, Foster NL, Fedio P (1984) Ann Neurol 15 (suppl.):175

8. Chiland C (1983) Neuropsych. Enfance 31(4):173-175

9. Cohen DJ, Shaywitz BA, Young JG et al (1978) Arch Gen Psychiatry 35: 245-250

10. Cohen DJ, Shaywitz BA, Young JG et al (1980) Arch Gen Psychiatry 37: 1350-1357

11. Comings DE, Gursey BT, Hecht T et al (1982) In: Friendhoff AJ, Chase TN

(eds) Gilles de la Tourette Syndrome. New York Press, pp 251-253

12. De Veaugh-Geiss J (1980) Neurology 30:562-563

13. Denkla MB, Bempored JR, Mackay MC (1976) JAMA 235:1349-1351

14. Devinsky O (1983) Arch Neurology 40:508-514

15. Eldridge R, Sweet R, Lake CR et al (1977) Neurology 27:115-124

16. Ferenczi S (1921) In: Hogarth (ed). Further contribution to the theory and theory of psychoanalysis

17. Ferrari E (1982) In: Atti VII Congresso Nazionale Società Italiana di Neuro pediatria

18. Freud S, Breuer S (1980) In: Boringhieri (ed) Opere. Torino

19. Gilles de la Tourette G (1985) Arch Neurol 9:19-42, 158-200

20. Gillies DRN, Forsythe WI (1984) Dev Med Child Neurol 26/6:830-833

21. Gonce M, Dugas M (1986) Encycl Med Chir (Paris France) Neurologie 17059C10: 12:5

22. Jankpvic J, Glaze DG, Frost JD (1984) Neurology 34:688-692

23. Kidd KK, Pauls DL (1982) In: Friendhoff AJ, Chase TN (eds) Gilles de la Tourette Syndrome Raven Press, New York, pp243-249

24. Kidd KK, Prusoff BA, Cohen DJ (1980) Arch Gen Psychiatry 37:1336-1339

25. Klawans HL, Falk DK, Nausieda PA et al (1978) Neurology 28:1064-1068

26. Klein M (1948) In: Hogarth(ed)

27. Kreisler L (1986) In: Cortina R (ed), Milano

28. Lebovici S (1952) In: PUF (ed) Paris   Les Tics Chez L'enfant

29. Lebovici S, Rabain JF, Nathan T et al (1986) Psichiatrie de l'enfant 1:5-59

30. Leckman JF, Cohen DJ, Detlor J et al (1982) In: Friedhoff AJ, Chase TN (eds) Gilles de la Tourette Syndrome. Raven Press, New York, pp391-401

31. Lucas AR, Beard CM, Rajput AH, Kurkland LT (1982) Adc Neurol 35:267-269

32. Mahler MS (1949) The Psychoanalitic study of the child 3/4:279-310

33. Marsden CD (1982) Lancet 2:1141-1142

34. Meige H, Feindel E (1902) In: Masson et C.ie (ed). Les tics et leurs traitments

35. Mueller J, Aminoff MJ (1982) Br J Psychiatry 141:191-193

36. Nee Le, Caine ED, Polinsky RJ et al (1980) Ann Neurol 7:41-49

37. Obeso JA, Rothwell JC, Marsden C (1981) J Neurol Neurosurg Psychiatry 44: 735-738

38. Polinsky RJ, Ebert MH, Caine ED et al (1980) N Engl J Med 302:1310

39. Rouart J (1947) Evolution Psychiatrique i; 86

40. Salami K (1961) Acta Psychiatr Scand 36:157-162

41. Scelkunov EL, Kenunen OG, Pushkov VV, Charitonov RA (1986) J Am Acad Child Psychiatry 25,5:645-652

42. Shapiro AK, Shapiro E, Sweet ED (1981) In: Barbeau A (ed) Disorders of movement. MT London, pp105-132

43. Shapiro AK, Shapiro E, Wayne H (1973) Arch Gen Psychiatry 28:92-97

44. Singer HS, Tune Le, Butler JJ et al (1982) Neurology 12:361-366

45. Tanner CM, Goetz CG, Klawans HL (1982) Neurology 32:1315-1317

46. Van Woert MH, Jutkowitz R, Rosembaum D, Bowers MB (1976) In: Yahr MD (ed) The basal ganglion. Raven Press, New York

© 1987 Elsevier Science Publishers B.V. (Biomedical Division)
Extrapyramidal disorders in childhood
L. Angelini et al. editors

WILSON'S DISEASE

ALDO CERNIBORI

Servizio di Neuropsichiatria Infantile,Ospedale Civile,23100 Sondrio,Italy

ISOLDA LA BUONORA

Servizio di Neuropsichiatria Infantile,Ospedale Civile,23100 Sondrio,Italy

ALBERTO OTTOLINI

Cattedra di Neuropsichiatria Infantile dell'Università,27100 Pavia,Italy

Wilson's disease(WD) is an infrequent hereditary disorder,not as rare as commonly thought,due to an inborn abnormality of copper metabolism leading to deposition of this metal in the central nervous system ,liver,cornea and kidney.Wilson(1) described the disease that bears his name in 1912;other cases as reported by Martin(2) had been previously seen by Westphal and Strümpell (3,4).In 1902 Kayser(5) draw attention to the typical corneal ring,described later by Fleischer(7).Cumings(7)in 1948 demonstrated deposition of copper in basal ganglia and liver.

The characteristic triad of WD consists of neurologic symptoms,hepatic cirrhosis and Kayser Fleischer corneal ring;most cases however initially show either neurologic or hepatic symptomatology.This can proceed so quickly that neurologic signs have no time to appear.The age of onset is from 7 to 15 years of age;some cases develop earlier than 2 years or later than 50 (8).

The juvenile form is characterized by a relatively quick evolution of signs, both hepatic (ascites,jaundice,hepatic coma) and neurologic (dysarthria,dysphagia,muscular spasms,rigidity,spasticity).In the late onset type,beginning between 20 and 30 years of age, the evolution is slower and the predominant neurologic symptom is the flapping tremor.

GENETICS

The inheritance of WD is autosomal recessive and the familial incidence is characteristic of the disorder.Thus,if a young person has liver cirrhosis,a sib presenting with jaundice or hemolytic anemia must be suspected as suffering from WD. The incidence of this disorder is stimated as 1 case in 200.000 births and its prevalence is 1 in 10.000. This estimate is surely far too low.Three clinical forms of the disease have been described and this fact has raised the possibility of three genetically heterogeneous disorders:1) a juvenile form,beginning before 15 years of age with predominant hepatic symptoms,affecting Western Europeans and Mediterranean ethnic groups; 2) a late onset,predominantly neurologic form,beginning after 20 years of age,affecting mainly Slavs and East Europeans;3) an atypical form,characterized by low serum ceruloplasmin in heterozigotes.We have personally observed the coexistence of different forms of WD in sibs.This fact make us question the heterogeneous genetic characteristics of the disease,that certainly bears further investigation.

PATHOLOGY

In the central nervous system basal ganglia,cortex,cerebellum and less often the corticospinal tracts are involved.In cases with neurologic symptoms the putamen is shrunken and degenerative changes can proceed to cavitation; small hemorrhages may also be present. Microscopically there is severe diminuition of nerve cells and loss of myelinated fibres ;cellularity however is diminution by an increase in glial cells. A characteristics pathologic feature of WD is the Opalski cell,large,round with coarsely granular cytoplasm and oval nucleus staining yellow brown with hematoxylin Van Gieson,found in the subthalamic nucleus,globus pallidus,thalamus and substantia nigra, and less frequently in the putamen,caudate and parietal cortex(9); copper deposits are present in the putamen.The liver is grossly nodular with fibrous bands;microscopically copper deposits are present and the liver shows a multilobular cirrhosis.Splenomegaly is usually secondary to cirrhosis.Cardiomegaly,due to a degenerative process of the myocardium or coronary vessels,indipendent of copper deposits, hepatic cirrhosis or chelating therapy has been observed.Descemet's membrane presents pigmented granules containing copper,giving rise to the gray or brown corneal ring,seen either with the slit lamp or with the naked eye.

CLINICAL FEATURES

WD affects many organs,thus the clinical features are highly variable.The number of patients appearing with the classic triad (neurologic manifestations, hepatic cirrhosis and corneal ring)is very small.The mode of onset,specially in children,can point to other diseases:hemolytic crisis with anemia and jaundice,bone lesions like those in Vitamin D resistent rickets(10).The progression of the disease can be either acute or chronic.Acute cases present generally with hepatic symptoms:vomiting,hemolysis,jaundice,ascites.Slowly evolving cases frequently manifest with school failure and lack of attention,dysarthria, slowing and slurring of speech.Some cases begin as reading disorders.Emotional disturbances and conduct disorders may erroneously point to a dissociative or neurotic form (11,12,13,14).

Two distinct types of neurologic involvement are recognized:a dystonic form with rigidity,spasticity,drooling of saliva,dysarthria,dysphagia and painful muscular spasms leading to contractures; and a pseudosclerotic,slowly evolving form,with flapping tremor of the wrists and shoulders.Clinically intermediate forms are frequently seen.

The facies is amimic,with a gaping smile due to retraction of the corners
of the mouth.There is inability to protrude the tongue.Dysarthria takes the
form of indistinct articulation,slowing or festination of speech: it can show
cerebellar,pseudobulbar or parkinsonian traits(15).Dysphonia may also be pre-
sent.Hypertonus,bradykinesia,presence of cogwheel phenomenon,characteristic
of extrapyramidal disease are observed,and occur in painful spasms or give
rise to fixed,abnormal positions.Walking is difficult,with loss of upper limbs
syncinesiae.Maintenance of erect posture and rising from a recumbent position
become impossible.Tremor can be parkinsonian or occur chiefly during movement;
it can also have the characteristics of asterixis. Occasionally epileptic seizures of jacksonian type or vertiginous attacks can develop.Pyramidal signs
are infrequent.An alteration of consciousness resembling Kretschmer apallic
syndrome can appear(9). Psychiatric involvement with personality disturbances
depression or euphoria are quite common.

Symptoms attributable to lever disease are jaundice,vomiting,hepatomegaly,
ascites. Kayser Fleischer ring is peculiar of this disease:it is a grey brown
ring on the cornea inner surface but it is not patognomonic being present in
other types of chronic liver disease too.

Involvement of other organs is less frequent:disturbance of renal function
with mild hematuria and proteinuria,endocrine dysfunction (amenorrhea,blood
sugar disorders),bone lesions with formation of cysts or osteoporosis and
pathologic fractures(10)

LABORATORY INVESTIGATIONS

Biochemical findings in WD are characteristic. The serum ceruloplasmin
level is generally lower than 10mg/100ml(normal values are 20-30mg/100ml.The
serum copper level is also lowered (less than 50 mcg/100 ml;normal values
are 85-100 mcg /100 ml);the non ceruloplasmin bound serum copper however is
elevated.Urinary copper is high,frequently reaching 100-1000 mcg/24 hours
(normal values are under 50 mcg/24 hours). Copper can be measured in liver
tissue obtained by needle biopsy.Copper content is increased in WD patients
and in heterozygous carriers;the normal value is about 10-20 mcg/100 g
dry weight;in WD patients this value is increased manyfold.

Electroencephalographic abnormalities are often seen in juvenile onset cases
of WD;Nevsimalova et al.(16) observed in 84% of recordings aspecific abnormalities;specific alterations are sometimes seen in heterozygous children of
mothers suffering from WD due to the toxic effects of copper during intrauterine life.The electroencephalographic abnormalities tend to improve
during D-penicillamine therapy.

Somatosensory,acustic and visual evoked potentials show a marked increase
of the peak latency(17).These abnormalities are not closely related to the
clinical course of the disease(18).Krause et al.(19) have studied acustic evoked
potentials in WD and have found abnormalities in two thirds of all cases.Vi-
sual evoked potentials improve during the course of D-penicillamine therapy;
reapeated VEP investigations allow monitoring of the therapeutic effect of
the drug(20).

Bone and joint radiographic investigations in WD demonstrate osteoporosis,
osteomalacia,bone cysts and pathologic fractures.

Computerized tomography(CT) show central nervous system and abdominal lesions
(21,22,23,24).Cortical atrophy,ventricular enlargement,low density areas lying
in the basal ganglia,cerebellum,brain stem and hemispheric white matter are
the most frequent images (25).CT lesions tend to improve during therapy with
chelating agents(26),but there is no close corrispondence between CT and clinical improvement(23,27).Low density areas are probably not due to copper
deposition but to structural modifications caused by edema(22).

Magnetic resonance (MR)imaging of the brain shows abnormalities of the lenticular and caudate nucleus,thalamus,red nucleus,substantia nigra and periacqueductal gray matter(22,28). MR has shown that while grey matter lesions
are usually symmetric,this is not true for the white matter abnormalities.
Uhlenbrock et al.(29) affirms that MR is preferable to CT in demonstrating
CNS lesions in WD.

TREATEMENT

If not suitably treated, WD is fatal in a matter of years.Effective therapy is now available with partial or complete remission of neurologic,ocular
and hepatic abnormalities.Numerous drugs had been proposed to treat WD:methioni-
ne,choline,corticosteroid drugs etc. In 1948 Cumings(17) suggested that the
use of BAL(2,3 dimercaptopropanolol) might remove copper from liver,brain
and other organs;BAL is a chelating agent with cupriuretic action.The dosage
is 2.5 mg/kg given by deep subcutaneous injection,twice a day,for one week;
after one week another course is administered.Thereafter 100-200 mg of BAL are
given every 15 days.

D-penicillamine (beta,beta dimethylcysteine) introduced in 1956(30) reduces
serum copper levels and enhances urinary copper excretion(31); this is also a
chelating agent with the big advantage of being administered by mouth,and
effective for long periods(32,33); recomended   dosage is 0.9-1.8 g/die.
D-penicillamine is a Vit.B_6 antagonist,so pyridoxin must be associated (B_6
50 mg/die); during pregnancy D-penicillamine must be given in lower dosage
to reduce a possible teratogenic risk(34). Clinical benefits parallel histo-

logic improvement of hepatic structure(35).Modai et al.(36) have pointed to
the disappearance of psychiatric symptoms with D-penicillamine therapy.Side
effects and toxic reactions due to this treatment are optic neuropathy,related
to Vit.B_6 deficiency,manifestations of hypersensibility(fever,skin rash,lympha-
denopathy,pancytopenia).Long term therapy can be complicated by a lupus ery-
thematosus-like syndrome and by retinal detachment during thrombocytopenia
(37,38).The development of nephrotic syndrome is another serious complication
of D-penicillamine therapy.

Another drug TETA (Triethylene tetramine dihydrochloride) has similar properties and can be introduced in case of D-penicillamine intollerance.The recommended dosage is 40-60 mg/kg/die (27).

Antiparkinsonian agents (L-dopa and Amantadine) are also utilized to allevia-
te extrapyramidal symptoms .Barbeau et al.(39),Gelmers et al.(40),Morgan et al.
(41) have reported their experience with the association L-dopa D-penicillami-
ne.L-dopa,500mg/day diminishes drooling,hypertonus,dysarthria and tremor.Aman-
tadine in association with L-dopa is also indicated.The recommended dosage is
200-400 mg/day(42).

Another approach to WD treatment is to reduce copper intake and its absorption
through an adequate diet and the utilization of zinc sulphate.A low copper diet
must exclude chocolate,liver,brain,seafood mushrooms and nuts.Zinc sulphate
blocks copper absorption in the gut.The dosage recommended is 50-100mg t.i.d.
in children less than ten years old and 200-300mg t.i.d. in older children
(43,44,45).In the gastrointestinal tract zinc induces the synthesis of metallothionein in the mucosal cells.Metallothionein binds copper that remains
blocked and ultimately will be lost by the normal desquamation of these cells.
The effect of zinc sulphate was demonstrated by oral administration of Cu^{64}
(46).In some cases with irreversibly liver damage not responding to drug therapy,liver transplantation has been suggested(24);Nazer et al.(47)have proposed guidelines to differentiate those WD patients who would benefit from a
liver transplantation

PATHOGENESIS

In spite of advances in understanding copper metabolism the primary error
in WD remains obscure.Among many working hypothesis two of them,diminuished
ceruloplasmin synthesis and presence of an intracellular protein with high
binding affinity to copper,are now actively investigated.

The daily supply of copper is 2-5 mg;the total amount of this metal in a normal adult is 75-150 mg.The highest concentrations are found in liver,brain
(locus ceruleus,substantia nigra),kidney and heart.A large amount of body copper

lies within the muscle mass.

Copper absorption in the gastrointestinal tract occurs largely from the stomach,duodenum and upper ileum.After passing the intestinal barrier copper is bound to albumin,one of the many protein carriers of this metal in the blood. In the liver copper is incorporated into an alpha $_2$ globulin,forming ceruloplasmin,another copper carrying protein that appears in plasma.Ceruloplasmin is a metalloprotein functioning as an enzyme as many other copper containing proteins(cytochrome oxidase,tyrosinase,monoamino oxidase,superoxide dismutase). The activity of ceruloplasmin is manyfold:regulation of copper absorption in the gut,synthesis of cytochrome oxidase(48),maintenance of normal levels of biogenic amines(49,50).The lack of modulation due to low levels of this substance explains the psychiatric disturbances in WD and the hallucinogenic effects of drugs inhibiting ceruloplasmin.In plasma copper is bound not only to albumin and ceruloplasmin,but also to aminoacids.Excretion of this metal occurs mainly through the fecal route(51),a fraction is lost by the kidney.In WD serum ceruloplasmin is low(less than 20 mg/100 ml),serum copper is also low (lower than 80 mcg/100 ml).Non ceruloplasmin bound copper instead is elevated and this fraction deposits in the tissues with toxic effects and is also excreted by the kidney. The fact that liver copper is bound to other substances,metallothionein and copper associated protein(CAP),has given rise to the hypothesis that an inborn error of these copper related proteins is at the root of this dismetabolism.

Metallothionein is a lysosomial protein,present in many tissues,as in liver; in the hepatocyte it accepts albumin-transported copper while in the intestinal mucosa,it blockes copper absorption(52).Porter (53)has pointed to the capability of metallothionein to polimerize producing an insoluble copper associated protein or CAP,easily excreted in the bile. In WD metallothionein does not polimerize,remaining as a monomer with very high copper affinity;therefore ceruloplasmin synthesis is then   diminished(54),toxic monomer accumulates in the hepatocyte leaking to the blood and arriving at other organs:brain, cornea,kidneys etc.(55).

Another pathogenetic hypothesis,points to the lack of a transferase needed to incorporate copper into ceruloplasmin and to transport the metal from lysosomes.This hypothesis agrees with Deiss et al.(56) clinical classification of WD in four stages. During the first stage WD is asymptomatic;there is an increase in liver copper and a saturation of the binding capacity of metallothionein.In the second stage copper leaks into serum as albumin bound copper; liver damage begins and hemolytic crises can be seen.The third stage is characterized by central nervous system involvement,Kayser Fleischer ring formation and biochemical abnormalities.In the fourth stage the full blown disease is present with the characteristic clinical triad and biochemical and histological alterations.

There are still many unknown facts in copper metabolism,both normal and in WD.The foregoing hypothesis highlight the direction of current experimental studies.

REPORT OF TWO CASES

We shall now briefly propose two cases of WD just to underline its many unusual features.

The first case is a 15 years old male admitted because of behaviour disorders. No one in his family had previously suffered from hepatic or neurologic disease. One year earlier this boy began to act "different"; he preferred not to go out and see his friends;his humor changed without apparent reason.On admission he was very anxious and passed through moments of elevated mood with hyperactivity to periods of weeping and deep sadness.The neurologic examination showed signs of extrapyramidal disorder: fixity of facial expression with stereotyped smile, dysarthria,plastic hypertonus,fine rythmic tremor of the upper limbs. The contemporary presence of extrapyramidal and psychiatric signs made us suspect and then confirm the presence of WD.

The second case is a 17 years old boy suffering from progressive dysarthria. At 15 years of age he began with a tonic stammer so disabling that he had to leave school.On admittance his speech was unintelligible.The neurologic examination showed dystonic posturing of the fingers with hyperextension of the first, and flexion of the second phalanx.The laboratory studies showed a compromission of hepatic and renal function.Two anamnestic elements were also considered: an hemolytic crisis that the boy presented 5 years earlier and the fact that a sister had died at 3 because of fulminating hepatitis. We interpreted these findings as due probably to WD,confirmed later by laboratory examination.

Both cases were treated with D-penicillamine with good clinical results.

Lastly, we would like to report some sentences included in Walshe's description (57) confirming the variability of the clinical manifestations of this disorder: "...the truth is that no two patients are ever quite the same; there is no such thing as a typical case of Wilson's disease".

REFERENCES

1. Wilson SA (1912) Brain 34:295-509

2. Martin GP (1968) In: Vinken PJ,Bruyn GW (eds) Handbook of Clinical Neurology. North Holland Publishing Co,Amsterdam 6,11:267-278

3. Westphal C (1883) Arch.Psychiat.Nervenkr.14:87-134

148

4. Strümpell A (1898) Dtsch.Z.Nervenheilk.12:115-149

5. Kayser B (1902) Klin.Mbl.Augenheilk.40:22-25

6. Fleischer B (1912) Dtsch.Z.Nervenheilk.44:179-201

7. Cumings JN (1948) Brain 71:410-415

8. Lüthy F (1931) Dtsch.Z.Nervenheilk.123:101-181

9. Miyakawa T, Murayama E, Tatesu S (1976) Acta Neuropath.35:235-241

10. Goldstein B, Pepin B (1979) In: EMC (Neurologie) Paris 17060,A10,12

11. Basquin M (1975) Rev.de Neuropsych.Infantile 23,34:195-200

12. Cartwright G (1978) The New England Journal of Medicine 298,24:1347-1350

13. Dening TR (1985) British Journal of Psychiatry 147:677-682

14. Hymant N, Phuapradit P (1979) Journal of Neurology Neurosurgery and Psychiatry 42:478-480

15. Berry W, Darley F, Aronson E, Goldstein N (1974) Journal of Speech and Hearing research 17:169-183

16. Nevsimalova S, Marecek Z, Roth B (1986) Electroenceph.and Cl.Neurophysiology 64:191-198

17. Nai Shin Chu (1986) Brain 109:491-507

18. Roach ES, Ford C, Spudis E, Riela A, McLean W, Gilliam G, Ball M (1985) J.Neurol.232:20-23

19. Krause T, Pankau WP, Wagner A, Loszner J (1984) Psychiatr.Neurol.Psychol. 36,9:545-550

20. Haman KU, Hellner KA, Muller A, Zschockes S (1985) Fortschr.Ophthalmol.82, 2:194-196

21. Ropper AH, Hatten HP, Davis KR (1979) Ann.Neurol.5,1:102-103

22. Aisen A, Martel W, Gabrielesen T, Glazer G, Young A, Hill G (1985) Radiology 157,1:137-141

23. Williams FIB, Walshe JM (1981) Brain 104:735-752

24. Walshe JM, Dixon AK (1986) The Lancet April 12:845-847

25. Selekler K, Kausu T, Zileli T (1981) Arch.Neurol.38,11:727-728

26. Nix WA, Ludwig G, Backmund H (1984) Nervenarzt 55,10:544-548

27. Lingam S, Wilson J, Nazer H, Mowat AP (1987) Neuropediatrics 18:11-12

28. Lawler GA, Pennock JM, Steiner RE, Jenkins WS, Sherlock S, Young IR (1983) J.Comput.Assist.Tomogr.7:1-8

29. Uhlenbrock D, Straube A, Beyer HK, Leopold HC (1985) Digit.Bild Diagn.5, 3:120-122

30. Walshe JM (1956) Am.J.Med.21:487-495

31. Landrieu P, Choulot J (1976) Arch.Franc.Péd.33:665-675

32. Walshe JM (1962) Arch.Dis.Chil.37:253

33. Walshe JM (1967) Brain 90:149-174

34. Puissan C, Mathieu M (1985) J.Génét.Hum.33,3-4:357-362

35. Grand RJ, Vawter GF (1975) The Journal of Pediatrics 86,6:1161-1170

36. Modai I, Karp L, Liberman V, Munitz H (1985) 173,11:698-701

37. Klepach GL, Wray SH (1981) Ann.Ophthalmol.1312:201-203

38. Muyagawa S, Yoshioka A, Hatoko M, Okuchi T, Sakamoto K (1987) 116:95-100

39. Barbeau A, Frisien H (1970) The Lancet 11:1180

40. Gelmers H, Troost J, Willemse J (1973) 3:453-457

41. Morgan JP, Preziosi TJ, Bianchine JR (1970) The Lancet 11:659

42. Berio A, Vento R, Di Stefano A (1973) Min.Ped.25:807-813

43. Hoogenraad TU, Koevoet R, De Ruyter K (1979) European Journal of Neurology 18:205-211

44. Van Caillie Bertrand M, Degenhart HJ, Wisser HK, Sinaasappel M, Bpouquet J (1985) Arch.of Disease in Childhood 60:656-659

45. Hoogenraad TU, Van der Hamer C, Van Hattum J (1984) British Medical Journal 298:273-276

46. Hill G,Brewerg Juni J, Prasad A, Dick R (1986) Am.J.Med.Sci.292,6:344-349

47. Nazer H, Ede R, Mowat A, Williams R (1986) Gut.27:1377-1381

48. Broman L (1967) In: Walaas O (ed) Proceedings of Nato Advanced Study Institute Drammen.Academic London pp 131-150

49. Barras BC, Coult DB,Pinder RM, Skeels M (1973) Biochem.Pharmacol.22:2891-2895

50. Osaki S, McDermott JA, Frieden E (1964) J.Biol.Chem.239:3570-3575

51. O'Reilly S, Weber PM, Oswald M, Shipley L (1971) Arch.Neurol.25:28-32

52. Bremner J (1980) In: Mills CF (ed) Bilogical roles of copper.Excerpta Medica, Amsterdam,pp 23-26

53. Porter H (1984) Biochem.Biophys.Res.Commun.56:661-668

54. Evans GW, Dubois RS, Hambidge KM (1973) Science 181:1175-1176

55. Fowler BA, Nordberg GF (1978) Toxicol.Appl.Pharmacol.46:609-623

56. Deiss A, Lynch RE (1971) Ann.Intern.Med.75:57

57. Walshe JM (1976) In: Vinken PJ, Bruyn GW (eds) Handbook of Clinical Neurology.North Holland Publishing Co,Amsterdam 27,16:379-410

© 1987 Elsevier Science Publishers B.V. (Biomedical Division)
Extrapyramidal disorders in childhood
L. Angelini et al. editors

NEURORADIOLOGY OF BASAL GANGLIA DISEASES IN CHILDREN AND ADOLESCENTS

MARIO SAVOIARDO, ANGELO PASSERINI and LUDOVICO D'INCERTI

Department of Neuroradiology, Istituto Neurologico "C. Besta", Via Celoria,

11, 20133 MILANO (ITALY)

The role of neuroradiology in the study of the degenerative diseases

of the central nervous system was extremely limited up to the early '70s.

Pneumoencephalography (PEG) was only able to rule out mass lesions or to

demonstrate atrophy. The only disease affecting the basal ganglia in

which a positive diagnosis was supported by specific

pneumoencephalographic abnormalities was Huntington's chorea, in which

PEG could demonstrate the atrophy of the head of the caudate nucleus with

flattening of the lateral margin of the frontal horn.

In the last 15 years, first computed tomography (CT) and more recently

magnetic resonance imaging (MRI) have allowed the in vivo demonstration

of the brain parenchyma. The principles of these two different

techniques are quite different and their ability in demonstrating

lesions is also different; even the normal anatomy can be better

demonstrated by MRI because of its unique ability to differentiate grey

from white matter.

With CT, the whole lentiform nucleus can be visualized because of its

different density from the internal and external capsules that separate

it from the head of the caudate nucleus, the thalamus and the insular

cortex. With MRI, within the lentiform nucleus the pallidum can be

separated from the putamen because of its different cellular component and its high content of myelinated fibers from which its name derives. This should result in slightly shorter T1 and T2 relaxation times of the pallidum versus the putamen. However, with high strength magnetic field of 1.5 Tesla, an important observation was made (1): with increasing age, the signal of the pallidum in T2-weighted images becomes remarkably less intense; this also happens in other areas such as the substantia nigra, the red and the dentate nuclei, and to a much lesser extent, in the subcortical temporal white matter and in most of the brain.

This loss of signal due to shortening of T2 relaxation time in high-strength magnetic field has been found to correlate with the distribution of iron as demontrated by Perls stain (1) (Fig 1).

This observation has opened a new field. Ferritin or ferric non-heme iron and possibly other paramagnetic metabolites (2,3) accumulate with an abnormal distribution in basal ganglia in some degenerative diseases such as Parkinson-plus syndromes, that include Shy-Drager syndrome and

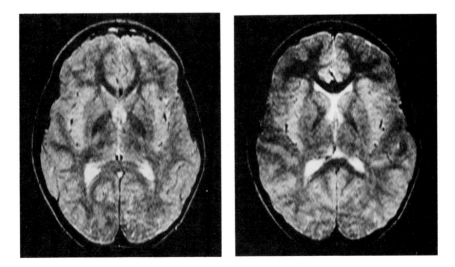

Fig. 1. T2-weighted images of normal basal ganglia. Low signal intensity in the pallidum is consistent with presence of ferric iron.

olivopontocerebellar degeneration, grouped under the term of "multisystem atrophies", and progressive supranuclear palsy. T2-weighted images obtained at high-strength magnetic fields may demonstrate, therefore, a loss of signal corresponding to an abnormally high concentration of iron in the putamen and in the pars compacta of the substantia nigra. In multisystem atrophies, the signal of the putamen, which is normally higher than that of the pallidum, becomes low, similar to or even lower than that of the pallidum.

How often this may happen in these diseases and what correlation may exist with the severity or with the duration of the disease have yet to be established. However, this finding may even become important in monitoring the effect of different therapies and illuminating results are expected in the next few years.

Most of these multisystem atrophies are diseases of old age and observations in young persons or children with, for instance, olivopontocerebellar degeneration, are not yet available. Hallervorden-Spatz disease is the only one of the age group that we are going to discuss, in which abnormal accumulation of iron in the basal ganglia is well known and in which the effects of iron on MRI images have been reported (4); this disease will be discussed in the appropriate section.

We shall now discuss the CT and MRI findings observed in the diseases affecting the basal ganglia in childhood and adolescence; we shall first consider the dystonic syndromes associated with hereditary neurologic disorders of probable metabolic degenerative origin; we shall then briefly discuss the non-hereditary dystonias caused by various intoxications or acute insults. We shall not therefore discuss all the primary,   idiopathic dystonias   in which neuroradiologic studies are

normal and we shall limit our discussion to the most frequently observed

disease and to those in which characteristic neuroradiological findings

have been observed.

DYSMETABOLIC OR DEGENERATIVE DISEASES AFFECTING THE BASAL GANGLIA IN
CHILDHOOD AND ADOLESCENCE

Wilson's disease

Wilson's disease is due to an inborn defect in the metabolism of

copper, that accumulates in basal ganglia and liver.

CT findings most frequently include mild atrophy and low density areas

in the basal ganglia, chiefly located in the putamina and the heads of

the caudate nuclei. Low attenuation areas, however, are sometimes present

in the thalamus (5) and questionably in the region of the dentate nuclei

(6). The lesions may be better demonstrated by MRI: they appear as a high

intensity signal in T2-weighted images in the same areas. Therefore, the

greater sensitivity of MRI may depict lesions not apparent on CT: an

abnormal signal may, therefore, also be demonstrated in the midbrain,

pons and subcortical white matter (7,8) In our 4 cases studied by MRI, an

abnormal signal was present in only the striatum in 3, and in the

striatum and thalami in the fourth.

Improvement in low density lesions seen on CT after treatment with chelating agents has sometimes been observed (9).

Leigh's disease (subacute necrotizing encephalomyelopathy)

This is an evolutive disease affecting mainly the basal ganglia, due to defects in the cytochrome-c-oxidase and or pyruvate dehydrogenase or other unidentified enzymes.

In Leigh's disease, CT findings of low density lesions in the putamina have been considered characteristic but have been observed in only 3 of our 8 cases. More recent reports emphasize the variability of CT findings even in this disease, with lucencies in the caudate and pallidum or even in white matter and cortical grey matter, with normal basal ganglia (10). Also in Leigh's disease MRI may show more extensive abnormalities than those demonstrated by CT. In addition to a low intensity signal in T1-weighted images and a high intensity signal in T2-weighted images in the putamina , MRI may show similar signal abnormalities in the brainstem, particularly in the periaqueductal region and in the pontine nuclei anterior to the floor of the fourth ventricle, in the heads of the caudate nuclei and in the periventricular white matter and cerebral cortex (11). Progression of the disease may modify the CT and MRI changes with the appearance of more extensive lesions and severe generalized atrophy (11).

156

Huntington's chorea

This is a hereditary disease of mendelian dominant type, mmanifested by choreiform movements and dementia. Only a small percentage of cases become manifest before age 15.

CT may support the diagnosis in early cases by demonstrating slight generalized atrophy with more focal enlargement of the frontal horns due to tissue loss in the heads of caudate nuclei. No abnormal densities are observed. MRI examination is often degraded by movement artifacts. However, of 3 patients examined with MRI - 2 adults and one 14-year-old girl - 2 with the rigid form of the disease (one adult and the girl) presented an abnormally elevated signal in T2-weighted images in the heads of the caudate nuclei and in the putamina, in addition to the usual focal atrophy (Fig. 2).

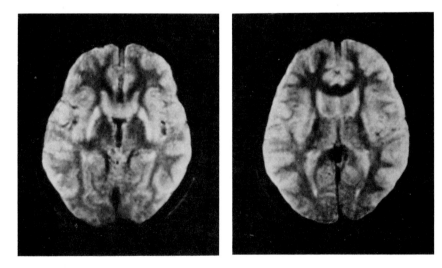

Fig. 2. Huntington's chorea, rigid form, in a 14-year-old girl. T2-weighted images show increased signal intensity in putamina and heads of caudate nuclei.

Dystonic syndromes associated with striatal CT low densities

In this chapter, several syndromes associated with various neurological disorders can be included.

The infantile bilateral striatal necrosis, as defined by Friede (12), is a variable progressive or acute disorder sometimes preceded by fever. In spite of neuronal loss and marked gliosis in the whole basal ganglia, CT may only show focal atrophy without density changes (13); however, lucencies in the putamina and heads of caudate nuclei have been observed (14). According to Goutières and Aicardi (14), it is likely that infantile bilateral striatal necrosis is a heterogeneous group of diseases, that includes cases of Leigh's disease, cases of familial degeneration of the striatum and cases of parainfections encephalitis that only affect the basal ganglia.

In reviewing patients with evolutive dystonias followed in our Institute, a group of 8 cases could be separated from the "idiopathic" dystonia cases that have normal neuroradiological studies (15). These 8 cases were characterized by low density lesions always affecting the putamina and sometimes also the heads of the caudate nuclei. MRI showed with greater evidence the same lesions but failed to show involvement of other areas. All biochemical investigations were normal. The only clinical difference between these cases and the idiopathic dystonias was that the children with lucencies in the neostriatum had a greater progression of their dystonia. Presence of CT or MRI striatal abnormalities in patients otherwise classifiable as idiopathic dystonia cases, may therefore indicate a worse prognosis and identify this not yet biochemically classified group (Fig. 3).

Other series of patients affected by **dystonia and Leber's optic atrophy**, or other forms of **visual failure** and characterized at CT by lucencies in the putamina have been reported (16,17). In the first group, associated with Leber's optic atrophy, later involvement of the caudate nuclei and of the thalami was also noted. Maternal non-mendelian cytoplasmic transmission and the possibility that the disease is a mitochondriopathy were also suggested on the consideration that the neostriatum is particularly sensitive to factors that inhibit mitochondrial enzymes, and that Leigh's disease and **Kearns-Sayre syndrome**, that are mitochondrial diseases, both exhibit putaminal lesions (16). In cases of striatal degeneration associated with Leber's optic atrophy, MRI confirmed the CT findings of lesions confined to the putamina occasionally involving the heads of caudate nuclei but without involvement of other structures of the central nervous system. The lesions, as usual, appeared as areas of low intensity signal in T1-weighted images and high intensity signal in T2-weighted images, consistent with increased water content (18).

Hallervorden-Spatz disease

This is an interesting disease to study with MRI, since it is known from neuropathology that, besides dysmyelination and atrophy, it involves abnormal iron storage in the lentiform nucleus, substantia nigra and red nucleus (4). Reports are scanty due to the rarity of the disease. In a case studied with a magnet operating at 0.15 Tesla, a low intensity signal in T1-weighted images and a high intensity signal in T2-weighted images in the basal ganglia were observed (19). However, in a case studied at 0.35 Tesla, the T2-weighted images demonstrated high intensity signal in the periventricular white matter, consistent with dysmyelination, but decreased signal in the lentiform nuclei (4). This may be interpreted as the paramagnetic effect of iron that, making locally inhomogeneous the magnetic field, causes a shortening of T2 relaxation time. The discrepancy between the two reports may be related to the different intensity of the magnetic fields, since the paramagnetic effect of iron is proportional to the square of the field intensity. In fact, we studied one adult patient with Shy-Drager disease (in which abnormal iron deposition in the putamen has been reported (2,3)) both with a 0.15 Tesla and a 1.5 Tesla units: in the first examination the putamen had a high signal in T2-weighted images, likely reflecting increased water content due to gliosis and/or cell loss; in the second examination, the putamen had a low signal probably reflecting the iron deposition effect which overcame the effect of water.

In one girl of 14 years of age with propable Hallervorden-Spatz disease, examined by us with a 1.5 Tesla magnet, a short T2 due to abnormal iron distribution was observed in the putamen, as well as in the pallidum (Fig 4).

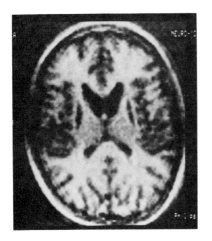 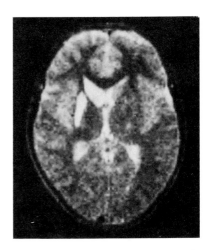

Fig. 3. Two different patients with evolutive dystonia. On the left low intensity signal is present bilaterally in the putamen and head of caudate nucleus in Inversion Recovery (T1 images). On the right, in a patient with unilateral dystonia, increased signal in T2-weighted images is present in the neostriatum on the opposite side.

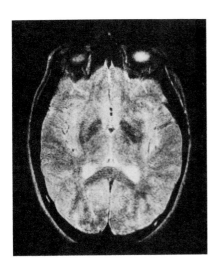

Fig. 4. T2-weighted image shows abnormally low signal in putamen, consistent with iron deposition, in a case of probable Hallervorden-Spatz disease.

Obviously, many more observations are needed to establish what the usual aspect of Hallervorden-Spatz disease will be.

Olivopontocerebellar degeneration

Olivopontocerebellar degeneration (OPCD) is a disorder of unknown etiology, occurring both in familial and sporadic cases, characterized by atrophy mainly of the cerebellum and brainstem.

CT often shows severe atrophic changes in posterior fossa. They may be present, to a lesser degree, in the cerebral hemispheres (20). OPCD is included in the multisystem atrophies and abnormal distribution of iron in the basal ganglia has been suggested (2). However, MRI performed with a 1.5 Tesla unit in a 10-year-old girl was normal except for the demonstration of atrophy in posterior fossa.

Other rare disorders affecting basal ganglia

Methylmalonic aciduria is an autosomal recessive disease due to methylmalonilCoA-mutase deficiency or related to vitamin B12 metabolism disorder, characterized by signs and symptoms of recurrent metabolic acidosis.

CT scan may show symmetrical low density lesions in the basal ganglia, confined to the pallidum, as we observed in one 5 year-old boy. Minimal enlargement of the frontal horns was also present.

Maple syrup urine disease (MSUD) is a familial metabolic disease in which an enzymatic defect causes accumulation of the branched chain aminoacids and their corresponding ketoacids.

Profound and diffuse changes in the white matter consistent with dysmyelination have been described. However, in a few of the reported cases, although not mentioned, and in a case we are reporting elsewhere (21), low density on CT and increased signal in T2-weighted images on MRI were also present in the pallidum, consistent with the spongiosis observed in this nucleus by Friede (12).

Finally, we should mention the **calcifications** that may occur in basal ganglia, particularly in the pallidum. There are familial forms, associated or not with various extrapyramidal disorders. The basal ganglia calcifications tend to be labelled as **Fahr's disease,** although this does not imply a better understanding of the disorder.

Calcifications in the basal ganglia are frequently observed in idiopathic hypoparathyroidism and in pseudohypoparathyroidism: their most common initial location is in the pallidum but they may extended to the putamen, caudate, thalamus, subcortical white matter and cerebellum in a symmetrical fashion (22). However, there are instances in which neither endocrine abnormalities, nor calcium metabolic disorders are detected: the significance of the basal ganglia calcifications in these cases remains unknown.

BASAL GANGLIA ABNORMALITIES DUE TO INTOXICATIONS OR OTHER ACUTE INSULTS

Ischemia and anoxia can cause bilateral lesions in the basal ganglia. Particularly perinatal asphyxia may cause lesions mainly located in the putamina that appear on CT as low density necrotic areas (23). The lesions may also extend to the heads of the caudate nuclei, and may obviously involve the thalami or other parts of the brain, depending on the length and severity of the anoxia.

Carbon monoxide (CO) intoxication and _cyanide poisoning_ also cause lesions in the basal ganglia as well as in other parts of the brain, probably identifiable as vascular watershed areas, in the surviving patients. Particularly cyanide is said to cause pallidal necrosis (24, 25), but a pathological report (26) as well as a case with MRI we observed indicate that the lesions involve both the pallidum and the putamen.

CONCLUSIONS

Several hereditary, metabolic diseases that affect the basal ganglia,
and anoxia and various intoxications may cause lesions detectable by CT
and even better by MRI.

There is little specificity in the appearance of all these lesions:
most of the hereditary, dysmetabolic disorders mainly affect the
neostriatum, while a few intoxications probably affect the pallidum more
frequently. When the neostriatum is involved, the putamen is always
affected; we have never observed lucencies or abnormal signals in the
heads of caudate nuclei without similar or more extensive lesions in the
putamina, while lesions in the putamina with normal caudate nuclei are
common. The cause of this susceptibility or vulnerability of the putamen
is unknown, but it may lie in different levels and distribution of
enzymes or metabolic processes. The answer to this question, however, can
not be given by the neuroradiologist, but by the biochemist of the
neurophysiopathologist.

The overlapping and the variability in the neuroradiological aspect of
these diseases is another factor that diminishes the possibility of a
specific diagnosis.

Generalizations from only a few observations may be hazardous and
misleading.

The importance of CT and MRI studies lies, therefore, in the demonstration that there is, indeed, a lesion in the basal ganglia, that, in the appropriate clinical setting, may support a specific diagnosis. On other occasions the lesion appears as a surprise and must lead to biochemical studies that are the only ones that may define these diseases.

The possibility of detecting iron or other paramagnetic metabolites by MRI will probably improve the diagnostic possibilities and will open new insights in some diseases and in their therapeutic approach.

ACKNOWLEDGEMENTS

We are grateful to Dr. Graziella Uziel and Dr. Nardo Nardocci for their helpful advice.

REFERENCES

1. Drayer B, Burger P, Darwin R, Riederer S, Herfkens R, Johnson GA (1986) Magnetic Resonance Imaging of Brain Iron. AJNR 7: 373-380

2. Drayer B, Olanow W, Burger P, Johnson GA, Herfkens R, Riederer S (1986) Parkinson Plus Syndrome: Diagnosis Using High Field MR Imaging of Brain Iron. Radiology 159: 493-498

3. Pastakia B, Polinsky R, Di Chiro G, Simmons JT, Brown R, Wener L (1986) Multiple System Atrophy (Shy-Drager Syndrome): MR Imaging. Radiology 159: 499-502

4. Littrup PJ, Gebarski SS (1985) MR Imaging of Hollervorden-Spatz Disease. J Comput Assist Tomogr 9: 491-493

5. Lawler GA, Pennock JM, Steiner RE, Jenkins WJ, Sherlocks, Young IR (1983) Nuclear Magnetic Resonance (NMR) Imaging in Wilson Disease. J Comput Assist Tomogr 7: 1-8

6. Kvicala V, Vymazal J, Nevsimalova S (1983) Computed Tomography of Wilson Disease. AJNR 4: 429-430

7. Aisen AM, Martel W, Gabrielsen TO, Glazer GM, Brewer G, Young AB, Hill G (1985) Wilson Disease of the Brain: MR Imaging. Radiology 157: 137- 141

8. Starosta-Rubinstein S, Young AB, Kluin K, Hill G, Aisen AM, Gabrielsen T, Brewer GJ (1987) Clinical Assessment of 31 Patients with Wilson's Disease. Correlations With Structural Changes of Magnetic Resonance Imaging. Arch Neurol 44: 365-370

9. Williams JB, Walshe JM (1981) Wilson's Disease - an Analysis of the Cranial Computerized Tomographic Appearances Found in 60 Patients and the Changes in Response to Treatment with Chelating Agents. Brain 104: 735-752

10. Paltiel HJ, O'Gorman AM, Meagher-Villemure K, Rosenblatt B, Silver K, Watters GV (1987) Subacute Necrotizing Encephalomyelopathy (Leigh Disease): CT Study. Radiology 162: 115-118

11. Davis PC, Hoffman JC Jr, Braun IF, Ahmann P, Krawiecki N (1987) MR of Leigh's Disease (Subacute Necrotizing Encephalomyelopathy). AJNR 8: 71-75

12. Friede RL (1975) Developmental neuropathology. Springer-Verlag, Wien

13. Mito T, Tanaka T, Becker LE, Takashima S, Tanaka J (1986) Infantile Bilateral Striatal Necrosis. Clinicopathological Classification. Arch Neurol 43: 677-680

14. Goutieres F, Aicardi J (1982) Acute Neurological Dysfunction Associated with Destructive Lesions of the Basal Ganglia in Children. Ann Neurol 12: 328-332

15. Nardocci N, Angelini L, Lamperti E, Rumi V, Savoiardo M (1986) Neostriatal Degeneration and Dystonic Syndromes of Childhood. International Symposium on Movement Disorders. Barcelona. Spain, 18-20 sept. 1986

16. Novotny EJ Jr, Singh G, Wallace DC, Dorfman LJ, Louis A, Sogg RL, Steinman L (1986) Leber's Disease and Dystonia: a Mmytocondrial Disease. Neurology 36: 1053-1060

17. Marsden CD, Lang AE, Quinn NP, McDonald WI, Abdallat A, Nimri S (1986). Familial Dystonia and Visual Failure with Striatal CT Lucencies. J Neurol Neurosurg and Psychiatry 49: 500-509

18. Seidenwurm D, Novotny EJ Jr, Marshall W, Enzmann D (1985) MR and CT in Cytoplasmically Inherited Striatal Degeneration. AJNR 7: 629-632

19. Johnson MA, Pennock JM, Bydder GM, Steiner RE, Thomas DJ, Hayward R, Bryant DRT, Payne JA, Levene MI, Whitelaw A, Dubowitz LMS, Dubowitz V (1983) Clinical NMR Imaging of the Brain in Children: Normal and Neurologic Disease. AJNR 4: 1013-1026

20. Savoiardo M, Bracchi M, Passerini A, Visciani A, Di Donato S, Cocchini F (1983) Computed Tomography of Olivopontocerebellar Degeneration. AJNR 4: 509-512

21. Uziel G, Savoiardo M, Nardocci N (1987) Computed Tomography and Magnetic Resonance Imaging in Maple Syrup Urine Disease. In preparation

22. Illum F, Dupont E (1985) Prevalence of CT-detected Calcification in the Basal Ganglia in Idiopathic Hypoparathyroidism and Pseudohypoparathyroidism. Neuroradiology 27: 32-37

23. Kretzschmar K, Ludwig B, Kramer G, Collmann H, Kazner E (1986) Bilateral Lesions of the Putamina. Neuroradiology 28: 87-91

24. Chi JG, Yoo HW, Chang KH, Kim CW, Moon HR, Ko KW (1981) Leigh's Subacute Necrotizing Encephalomyelopathy: Possible Diagnosis by CT Scan. Neuroradiology 22: 141-144

25. Finelli P (1981) Changes in the Basal Ganglia Following Cyanide Poisoning. J Comput Assist Tomogr 5: 755-756

26. Uitti RJ, Rajput AH, Ashenhurst EM, Rozdilsky B (1985) Cyanide-induced Parkinsonism: A Clinicopathologic Report. Neurology 35: 921-921

PHARMACOLOGICAL TREATMENT OF DYSTONIA

NARDO NARDOCCI, ELENA LAMPERTI, LUCIA ANGELINI

Department of Child Neurology, Istituto Neurologico "C. Besta", 20133 Milano (Italy)

INTRODUCTION

The pharmacological treatment of the patients with Dystonia is frequently very difficult. In some aetiological forms of Dystonia, as in drug-induced dystonia, a specific treatment is available. Dystonia, due to anticonvulsants can be treated by reducing the dosage of the drug and dystonic reactions secondary to antipsychotic drugs can respond to the administration of anticholinergics. In the majority of patients with either Idiopathic or Symptomatic Dystonia conversely only a non specific treatment is available. This therapy in part addresses itself to treat the symptoms but not the causes of the disease.

Moreover, the patients with these disorders do not show any consistent pharmacological response to the different classes of drugs that have been tried and it is impossible to predict which patients would benefit from which drug and which wouldn't benefit at all. This condition is due to numerous factors and we will now attempt to identify the most significant ones.

1) Idiopathic Dystonia is a non homogeneous disorder including hereditary and early onset forms with various modes of transmission ; sporadic late forms; focal, segmental and generalized forms; dystonia associated with other neurological disturbances such as tremor and Parkinsonian symptoms.

2) Biochemical neuropathology of idiopathic dystonia is unknown. No consistent neuropathological abnormalities have been observed in the brain of patients who have died with idiopathic dystonia (1, 2). No information is available regarding the basic neurochemical abnormality in idiopathic dystonia (3).

Many studies have reported about putative neurotransmitters or their metabolites in the cerebrospinal fluid of patients with idiopathic dystonia.

No abnormality was found in the level of GABA or glutamic acid in spinal fluid (4) or in the level of homovanillic acid or hydroxyindoleacetic acid in ventricular fluid (5, 6).

A reduction of lumbar CSF tetrahydrobiopterin (a co-factor for tyrosin hydroxylase) level in patients with various types of dystonia has been reported (7, 8).

On the basis of biochemical studies of the brains of two patients with generalized childhood onset dystonia, it has been recently hypothesized that a disturbance of noradrenergic brain mechanism represents the basic neurochemical abnormality of this disorder (2).

These data seem to support the previous report of a significant reduction of norepinephrine metabolite MHPG in the ventricular fluid of nine patients with childhood onset dystonia (9).

3) Until a few years ago, the majority of clinical pharmacological studies referred to a few cases and the results of treatment have been assessed by arbitrary and subjective evaluation.

In conclusion, the choice of treatment is not based on reliable rational criteria but, rather, on empirical data that are the results of clinical experience.

In the last few years, however, there have been numerous studies on a large group of patients which have thus furthered existing knowledge in the formulation of some therapeutic criteria.

Pharmacotherapy

The following review does not include every drug treatment carried out on dystonic patients, but focuses on those drugs that have shown a significant efficacy in a certain number of patients.

This review, moreover, addresses itself to the treatment of childhood onset dystonia and is limited to the drugs for systemic administration. It does not include the local administration of botulinum toxin which is used only in focal dystonia in adults.

Finally, the review is organized by classes of drugs.

Dopamine agonist

After the introduction of L-Dopa in the treatment of Parkinson's disease, this drug was also tried in patients suffering from idiopathic dystonia.

Investigations have not found significant abnormality of CNS dopamine or other monoamines, but other evidence indirectly implicates dopaminergic pathways in dystonia: lesions of the dopamine rich neostriatum can cause dystonia, as can acute administration of dopamine-blocking drugs; Parkinsonian patients, who have a nigro neostriatal dopamine deficiency may also show dystonic features and develop dystonia as a side effect of levodopa treatment.

Results of this drug however appeared contradictory: a favorable response (10, 11), no particular benefit (12, 13, 14) or a deterioration of symptoms have been reported (15).

The efficacy of L-Dopa and other dopamine agonist drugs have been subsequently evaluated in several studies. A recent review (16) points out that only few patients benefited from this class of drugs. Among Dopamine agonist drugs, both Bromocriptine (17,18,19,20) and Lisuride (21,22) have practically the same efficacy in comparison with L-Dopa.

Instead a variant of hereditary generalized dystonia characterized by marked diurnal fluctuation represents a sure indication for treatment with low doses of L-Dopa or Dopamine agonists (23, 24, 25). In these patients the highly positive efficacy of treatment does not decrease during long term treatment (26).

In those few L-Dopa responsive patients, the benefits are usually impressive. A recent study reports that about 10% of the patients with childhood onset dystonia with or without diurnal fluctuation responded dramatically to this drug (27). In accordance with the Authors these patients have to be considered affected by a variant of idiopathic dystonia.

As a result of this potential efficacy it is advised that L-Dopa therapy must be the initial treatment for all patients with childhood onset dystonia (28).

Dopamine antagonists

It is interesting to consider that one group of dystonic patients have a favorable response to Dopamine agonists, while an other group, suffering from the same disease, can likewise be responsive to other drugs with an opposite action, such as Dopamine receptor blockers and Dopamine storage depletors.

A possible explanation for this response is that idiopathic dystonia can have different pathogenetic mechanisms: the fact that no patient has been documentated as responding in the same way to both drugs strengthens this hypothesis.

The most widely used drugs in this category are phenotiazines, haloperidol, pimozide and tetrabenazine. As for the other classes of drugs, the efficacy in a single patient is variable and unpredictable (29).

With respect to Dopamine agonists the results are more constant, notwithstanding the fact that the side effects are more frequent (30,31,32,33,34).

Considering the incostant efficacy and the incidence of side effects, this class of drugs must never be considered as the first choice of treatment, particularly in young patients. The use of Dopamine antagonists must be reserved for those patients who do not respond to Dopamine agonists and anticholinergics (28).

Often, in clinical practice, when it is impossible to reduce the dystonic symptoms using only one drug, a combined therapy is necessary. Positive results in spasmodic torticollis and in axial dystonia (35) with a combined therapy of pimozide and trihexyphenidyl have been reported. An association of three drugs constituted by a low dose of Dopamine depletor (Tetrabenazine), plus a Dopamine receptor blocker (Pimozide) plus an anticholinergic (Triexiphenydile) has been proposed. This combined treatment was effective in the most severe cases (36).

Combined therapy may be administered to children, but it is not always advisable, because chronic dopaminic antagonist therapy can produce tardive dyskinesia. Therefore, it seems preferable to reserve this combined therapy for patients with more severe symptoms and/or for those extremely disabled.

Anticholinergic

Recently, numerous pharmacological studies of anticholinergic drugs have shown that this class of drugs offers the most consistent results.

First studies with low doses of anticholinergic (generally trihexyphenidyl) had already shown some validity in a variable percentage of patients (37,38,39,40), but it has generally been proven that a more constant improvement is evident with a high dose treatment (41, 36).

These results have also been confirmed in a double blind study (42). All these studies show that about 50% of childhood onset dystonia and 40% of adult patients respond positively to this class of drugs. A recent study on long-term anticholinergic treatment confirms such results, suggesting a correlation between the response and the duration of the disease before anticholinergic medication. Therefore the delay of treatment appears to be an unfavorable factor (43).

The main problem of anticholinergic treatment is the occurrence of adverse effects which dictates the limitation of dosage.

The more frequent adverse effects are dry mouth, and blurred vision (peripheral effects); confusion, hallucination and behavioural disturbances (central effects). These symptoms, however, usually disappear reducing the dosage.

Children tolerate high doses of anticholinergic better than adults. In the former high doses of trihexyphenidyl up to and over 80 mg/day can be administered, slowly increasing the dosage (40,41,42). Therefore, an initial dosage of 2.5 mg once or twice daily and an increase of 2.0 or 2.5 mg daily every one or two weeks is advised until the dystonia is controlled or side effects appear (28).

The mechanism and the site of the therapeutic effects of a high dose anticholinergic treatment in torsion dystonia is unknown.

A recent report suggests that the therapeutic efficacy is not due to the correction of a primary abnormality of cholinergic neurons in the striatum, but to a reduction of a functional over activity of the cholinergic brain mechanisms (2).

However, why a high dosage is necessary and the benefits are often delayed is not clear.

Other drugs

In the existing literature there are some reports on the efficacy of other drugs in the treatment of torsion dystonia, but generally the results are contradictory and variable.

The reports on Carbamazepine show that only a small percentage of patients responds to this drug (44, 45, 43).

The effectiveness of Benzodiazepines in cranial dystonia has been described (34). A recent report refers some efficacy of Clonazepam and other Benzodiazepines in 15% of 177 patients with various types of idiopathic dystonia. The same study reveals that 20% of the patients treated with Baclofen showed improvement (43).

No benefits were found in patients with dystonia to whom a GABAmimetic agent (the gamma vinyl GABA experimental drug), was administered (46). The Tetrahydrobiopterin (BH4) has been transiently effective in four out of eight dystonic patients (47).

CONCLUSIONS

From the analysis of the above reports it is possible to formulate certain therapeutic criteria in the treatment of the patients with idiopathic dystonia.

In accordance with Fahn and Marsden (28) the use of L-Dopa with inhibitor as the initial treatment is advisable. Already we have stated that some patients, particularly in childhood, can dramatically respond to this drug. The advised dosage is variable from 50 mg to 750 mg daily over a two month period.

The second choice is represented by an anticholinergic drug: of this class of drugs trihexyphenidyl is the most widely used; mention must be made again of the often delayed benefits of this treatment.

In those cases in whom no improvement or insufficient relief of symptoms have been achieved, the dose may be increased until the appearance of side effects.

When anticholinergic demonstrates some benefits but the dosage can not be increased, a combined therapy may be appropriate.

Proven differences in efficacy among Benzodiazepine, Carbamazepine or Baclofen have not been reported. Our experience, however, indicates a preference in the use of Benzodiazepines in young patients with dystonia secondary to brain injury or metabolic diseases.

In cases of failure, a treatment with a dopamine antagonist drug may be chosen, but the possible effects of long term administration of this class of drugs must be considered. The use of dop depletor, like Reserpine, in comparison with a dop receptor antagonist, seems to be preferable.

In concluding this review, we must emphasize that the aim of the pharmacotherapy is not to eradicate dystonia, but to restore the motor function. In patients with good autonomy it is preferable not to prescribe any drug therapy. When drugs are necessary, the gradual increase of the dosage is recommendable, allowing time to assess the highest efficacy using the lowest dosage.

This procedure is of particular importance in the use of the triheyphenidyl. In fact, as mentioned above, there is a low incidence of dose limiting side effects in childhood. The recognition, however, of the involvement of cholinergic mechanisms in intellectual performances underlines the possible consequences of this treatment.

REFERENCES

1. Zeman W (1970) Neurology 20: 79-88
2. Hornykiewicz O, Kish SS, Becker LE, Farley I, Shannak K (1986) N Engl J Med 315: 347-353
3. Bruyn GW, Roos RAC (1986) In: Vinken PS, Bruyn GW, Klawans HL (eds) Handbook of Clinical Neurology Vol 5. Elsevier, Amsterdam, pp 519-528
4. Perry TL, Hansen S, Quinn N, Marsden CD (1982) J. Neurochem 39: 1188-1191
5. Tabbador K, Wolfson LI, Sharpless NS (1978) Neurology 28: 1249-1253
6. Tabbador K, Wolfson LI, Sharpless NS (1978) Neurology 28: 1254-1258
7. Williams A, Eldridge R, Levine R (1979) Lancet II: 410-411
8. Lewitt PA, Miller LP, Levine RA (1986) Neurology (Cleveland) 36: 760-764
9. Wolfson LI, Sharpless NS, Thal LS (1983) Neurology 33: 369-372
10. Chase TN (1970) Neurology 20: 122-130
11. Coleman M (1970) Neurology 20: 114-121
12. Barrett RE, Yahr MD, Duvoisin RC (1970) Neurology 20: 122-130
13. Mandell S (1970) Neurology 20: 103-106
14. Eldridge R, Kanter W, Koerber T (1973) Lancet II: 1027-1028
15. Cooper IS (1972) Lancet II: 1317-1318
16. Lang AE (1985) Clin Neuroharmacol 8: 38-57
17. Sabouraud P, Allain H, Pinel JF, Menault F (1978) Nouv Press Med 7: 3370
18. Stahl SN, Berger PA (1982) Neurology 32: 889-892
19. Gautier JC, Awada A (1983) Rev Neurol (Paris) 139: 449-450
20. Newman RP, Lewitt PA, Shults C, Bruno G, Foster NL, Chase TN (1985) Clin Neuropharmacol 8: 328-333
21. Nutt JG, Hammerstad JP, Carter JH, De Garmo PL (1985) Neurology 35: 1242-1243
22. Quinn NP, Lang AE, Sheehy MP, Marsden CD (1985) Neurology 35: 766-769
23. Segawa M, Hosaka A, Miyagawa F, Nomura Y (1976) In: Eldridge K, Fahn S (eds) Advances in Neurology Vol 14, pp 215-233
24. Rondot P, Ziegler M (1983) J Neural Trasm Suppl 19: 273-281
25. Deonna T (1986) Neuropediatrics 17: 81-85
26. Segawa H, Nomura Y, Kase M (1986) In: Vinken PJ, Bruyn GW, Klawans H (eds) Handbook of Clinical Neurology Vol 5. Elsevier, Amsterdam. pp 529-539
27. Nygaard TG, Marsden CD, Duvoisin RC (1987) cited in: Marsden CD, Fahn S (eds) Movement Disorders 2. Butterworths, London
28. Fahn S, Marsden CD (1987) In: Marsden CD, Fahn S (eds) Movement Disorders 2. Butterworths, London, pp 359-382
29. Lang AE (19) cited in: Marsden CD, Fahn S (eds) Movement Disorders 2. Butterworths, London
30. Marsden CD (1981) In: Barbeau A (ed) Disorders of Movement. MPT Press Ltd,

176

Lancaster, pp

31. Jankovic J (1982) Ann Neurol 11: 41–47
32. Lang AE, Marsden CD (1982) Clin Neuropharmacol 5: 375–387
33. Girotti F, Scigliano G, Nardocci N, Angelini L, Broggi G (1982) J Neurol 33: 1255–1261
34. Jankovic J, Ford J (1983) Ann. Neurol 13: 402–411
35. Marsden CD, Fahn S (1982) In: Marsden CD, Fahn S (eds) Movement Disorders. Butterwoths, London, pp 191–195
36. Marsden CD, Marion MH, Quinn N (1984) J Neurol Neurosurg Psychiatry 47: 1166–1173
37. Marsden CD, Harrison MJG (1974) Brain 92: 793–810
38. Lal s, Hoyte K, Kiely ME, Soukkes TL (1979) Adv. Neurol 24: 335–351
39. Tanner CM, Goetz CS, Weiner WS, Nausieda PA, Wilson R, Klawans HL (1979) Neurology 29: 604–605
40. Marsden CD, Lang AE, Sheehy MP (1983) Neurology 33: 1100–1101
41. Fahn S (1983) Neurology 33: 1255–1261
42. Burke RE, Fahn S, Marsden CD (1986) Neurology 36: 160–164
43. Greene PE, Shale H, Fahn s (1987) cited in: Marsden CD, Fahn S (eds) Movement Disorders 2. Butterworths, London
44. Geller M, Kaplan B, Christoff N (1976) Advances in Neurology 14:403–410
45. Isgreen WP, Fahn S, Barrett RE, Snider SR, Chutorian AM (1976) Advances in Neurology 14: 411–416
46. Carella F, Girotti F, Scigliano C, Caraceni T, Joder-Ohlenbusch AM, Schechter PJ (1986) Neurology 36:98–100
47. Lewitt PA, Miller LB, Levine RA (1986) Neurology (Cleveland) 36: 760–764

© 1987 Elsevier Science Publishers B.V. (Biomedical Division)
Extrapyramidal disorders in childhood
L. Angelini et al. editors

SURGICAL TREATMENT OF DYSTONIAS AND OTHER ABNORMAL MOVEMENTS IN CHILDHOOOD

GIOVANNI BROGGI*, LUCIA ANGELINI**, NARDO NARDOCCI**, DOMENICO SERVELLO*, STEFANO CALDERINI**

*Dept. Neurosurgery and ** Dept. Child Neurology, Istituto Neurologico "C. Besta" 20133 Milano (Italy)

Functional neurosurgery - Definition and history

The Functional Neurosurgery is the performance of a lesion in certain, defined, brain structures in order to obtain a modification of pathological motor behavior.

The progression in our understanding of human neurophysiological mechanisms, combined with the development of more refined equipment for recording the electrical activity of the nervous system and for stimulating the nervous structures, has resulted in increasingly effective neurosurgical treatment of such conditions as movement disorders, pain and intractable epilepsy.

Neurosurgery in the early years focused on the treatment of lesions. With this growing knowledge of neurophysiological processes, surgery became involved also in the treatment of symptoms of underlying lesions, that do not require treatment or are untreatable.

Surgical therapy of abnormal movements, introduced by Horsley in 1909 (1), has carried out, for many years, ablative lesions of the motor cortex, of the pyramidal tract or of the cerebral peduncle. The principle of lesioning the corticospinal pathway to relieve motor disorders was based on the concept that this tract is the "final" motor pathway from the cerebral hemispheres to the spinal cord and that the prevalent output from the basal ganglia is directed to the premotor areas of the cortex through the thalamus.

Surgical lesioning of deep structures of the brain initiated, in 1940, by Meyers (2), as lesion of the caudate nucleus and globus pallidus.

Stereotactic neurosurgery was born, in 1906 from Clarke's original idea to reach the deep structures of the brain applying a cartesian tricoordinate system (3). By this method, calculations could be made and any point could be described by its coordinates. This technique reached a climax when Horsley and Clarke (1908) devised their so-called stereotactic apparatus. But it took nearly four decades until this technique, confined in experimental brain research on laboratory animals, was applied to the human brain, even if Clarke had anticipated the therapeutic possibilities of his invention in human neurosurgery.

A possible explanation can be the differences of variability between the skull of cats and monkeys and of humans. In the former, the coordinates of deep targets may be almost exactly determined in relation to reference points on the skull for its relative constance. In man these reference points appeared to be less sure because of their variability.

The application of this procedure in humans became possible using intracerebral reference points by x-ray contrast visualization of the ventricles (4, 5).

The first stereotactic operations on humans performed, in 1950, by Spiegel and Wycis, were coagulations of the globus pallidus, its efferent pathways, or the ansa lenticularis for the relief of parkinsonian tremor.

Cooper introduced the chemopallidectomy (stereotactic injection of alcohol and procaine in the pallidum) (8).

On the basis of anatomical evidence that the pallidum primarily projects to the thalamus, Hassler, in 1955 (9) proposed as a target of stereotactic lesions, the VL nucleus of the thalamus and Riechert carried out the first thalamotomy. Cooper, soon after, substituted the chemothalamectomy to the chemopallidectomy (10) Since its introduction, this surgical procedure has been performed, for many years, in the treatment of parkinsonian tremor.

In 1969 (11), Cooper extended the indication of this surgery to the patients with torsion dystonia and, in 1976, he reported, on the follow-up of 226 dystonic patients very favourable results (12). However, other neurosurgeons such as Mundinger (13), Riechert (14), Andrew (15) have reported no such benefits.

More recently, peripheral surgical methods for the treatment of focal dystonias (blepharospasm and spasmodic torticollis) have been proposed. These procedures are based on the extirpation or denervation of excessively contracting muscles (16-23).

The same principle underlines the local injection of botulinum toxin (24, 25).

Cervical cord stimulation was proposed, in 1982, by Waltz (26) and considered quite effective in the treatment of generalized and focal dystonias. A recent evaluation of this technique, verified in a double blind study, did not confirm these positive results and the procedure of stimulation has not yet been proposed (27).

Surgery of abnormal movement in childhood

In childhood, because of the high prevalence of bilateral or unilateral distribution of abnormal movements and the rarity of focal signs, the only surgical procedure is represented by stereotactic thalamotomy (28).

This surgery is based on the following anatomophysiological evidences. The ventral lateral and ventral anterior nuclei are specific nuclei related to the motor system. The ventral lateral nucleus receives input from the cerebellum (originated from the contralateral dentate nucleus and passed through the brachium conjuctivum) and projects to the motor cortex of the precentral gyrus.

The ventral anterior nucleus receives input from the globus pallidus, the efferent part of the Basal Ganglia. The projections to the thalamus from the globus pallidus are conveyed by two fiber bundles, the ansa lenticularis and the lenticular fasciculus; these two bundles later fuse together and reach the thalamus in the thalamic fasciculus. The projections from VL are directed to the premotor cortex of the frontal lobe, which lies rostral to the primary motor area.

The Basal Ganglia and the cerebellum constitute major subcortical reentrant loops of the motor system; they both receive input from the cerebral cortex and both project back to the cortex via the thalamus.

These nuclei have been chosen as surgical targets because the lesions induce an alteration of the input to the motor cortex.

VL and VA nuclei are identified in the anglosaxon literature and refer to the philogenetic scale. In german terminology (29) VL is subdivided into Voa (Ventralis oralis anterior) and Vop (Ventralis oralis posterior), when Voa includes part of VA. The more rostral part is identified as L.po (Latero polaris). This definition is usually adopted to describe the targets of the thalamotomies.

The literature on the efficacy of stereotactic thalamotomy in childhood is quite extensive (30-37), but the reports present a variable percentage of benefit, because of the difference of the indications for surgical treatment and no uniformity and assessment of pre and postoperative motor functions.

TABLE I

SUMMARY OF THE CASES

PT	AGE	SEX	CLINICAL FINDINGS		IMPROVEMENT
1	16	F	◑	D	++
2	12	F	◐	D	++
3	16	F	◑	D	++
4	19	F	◐	D	+++
5	18	M	●	D	±
6	19	M	◐	D	±
7	14	M	●	D	±
8	19	M	◑	D	+
9	12	M	◑	D	±
10	15	M	◐	D	+++
11	16	M	◑	D	+++
12	19	M	●	D	++
13	13	F	◑	D	++
14	14	M	◑	D	+++
15	14	F	●	D	+++
16	17	M	●	D	+++
17	15	M	◐	D	++
18	10	M	●	D	+++
19	17	M	●	D	++
20	13	M	●	D	+++
21	18	F	●	D	+
22	9	F	◑	D	+++

● Bilateral symptoms
◑◐ Unilateral symptoms
D = Dystonia   T = Tremor   H = Hyperkinesia

TABLE II

PT	AGE	SEX	CLINICAL FINDINGS		IMPROVEMENT
1	13	M	◖	Dt	+++
2	11	F	◑	Dt	+
3	15	F	●	Dt	+
4	18	F	◑	Dt	+++
5	13	F	◑	Dt	+++
6	19	M	●	Dt	+++
7	18	F	●	Dt	++

● Bilateral symptoms
◐◑ Unilateral symptoms
D = Dystonia   T = Tremor   H = Hyperkinesia

Moreover, a difficulty in evaluating the results of such surgery depends on the frequent discrepancy between the disappearance of abnormal movements and a real addiction of functional capacities.

Our intention is to specify the indications for surgical treatment of abnormal movements in childhood. The proposed criteria derived from the analysis of the surgical results of 46 patients who underwent stereotactic thalamotomy, from 1976 to the present in the Istituto Neurologico "C. Besta" of Milan (38, 39). The age of the patients ranges from 9 to 19 years (mean 14.8); the follow-up ranges from 1 to 7 years (mean 5).

The characteristics of the patients are summarized in table I, II, III.

As shown in table IV, 28 patients had bilateral motor signs: dystonic and/or hyperkinetic tetraparesis in the 23 cases of Cerebral Palsy and generalized dystonia in the 5 cases of Idiopathic Dystonia. In 18 cases the symptomatology was unilateral: dystonic and/or hyperkinetic hemiparesis in the 10 cases of Cerebral Palsy, segmentary dystonias in the 2 cases of Idiopathic Dystonia, and hemidystonias in the 4 cases secondary to vascular brain injury and in 2 cases secondary to head trauma.

The more disabling symptom, addressed to surgery, was represented by dystonia (dystonic movements and/or postures) in 28 cases, combined with action tremor in 8 cases, and by proxymal rapid hyperkinesia of large excursion in 17 cases.   In several patients with Cerebral Palsy, 19 in number, the abnormal movements were associated with spasticity.   38 patients underwent unilateral thalamotomy and 8 patients bilateral thalamotomy (2 patients during the same operation and the others in subsequent operations, with an interval of almost six months from each other; 1 patient had 4 subsequent operations).   In the majority of patients the operation has been carried out under local anesthesia; only a few cases, more severe, underwent general anesthesia.

TABLE III

PT	AGE	SEX	CLINICAL FINDINGS		IMPROVEMENT
1	12	M	●	H	++
2	13	F	●	H	+
3	14	F	●	H	+
4	18	F	●	H	−
5	11	M	●	H	±
6	15	F	●	H	++
7	15	F	●	H	+++
8	13	M	●	H	±
9	11	M	●	H	±
10	15	M	●	H	+
11	16	F	●	H	+
12	15	M	●	H	+
13	14	F	●	H	+
14	14	M	◐	H	+
15	13	F	●	H	+
16	12	F	●	H	+++
17	9	F	●	H	++

● Bilateral symptoms
◐◑ Unilateral symptoms
D = Dystonia   T = Tremor   H = Hyperkinesia

The surgical technique and choice of targets are presented in detail in a previous paper (39).

It must be noted that , in the first thalamotomies, the Lateral thalamotomy (VL; i.e. Voa, Vop and ZI) was combined with the Posterior one (Pulvinar-LP). This latter, in fact, was considered to be effective especially in the correction of the dystonias. Later, the posterior thalamotomy, in accordance with more recent morphofunctional data on the Complex Pulvinar-LP and the critical review of the clinical results, has not yet been performed (40, 41).

TABLE IV

DISTRIBUTION OF SYMPTOMS

BILATERAL	28	* Dystonic or hyperkinetic tetraparesis secondary to perinatal brain injury
		* Generalized Idiopathic Dystonias
UNILATERAL	18	* Dystonic or hyperkinetic hemiparesis secondary to perinatal brain injury
		* Segmentary Idiopathic Dystonias
		* Hemidystonia symptomatic of vascular and traumatic injury

Table V indicated the targets of surgery in our patients. The reported follow-up refers to the clinical status after the last operation of those patients who have had more than one operation.

All of the patients underwent, pre and postoperatively (15 days, 6 months, 1 year and subsequently every year) standard neuroradiological examination and functional evaluation with videotape recording. Functional status has been assessed by the following tests (42, 43).

1. The cerebral palsy assessment of Seemans is made up 20 items and evaluates postural control from the horizontal to the erect position.

2. The grasp test evaluates the ability to grasp three objects of different sizes.

3. The test to assess the autonomy in feeding and dressing explores the performance of overall movements in various every day activities.

4. The Siegfried and Perret' test studies the precision of movements of the upper limb by means of tracing.

This evaluation has been extended not only to the patients with cerebral palsy, but also to others with secondary dystonias and to the few cases with idiopathic dystonia. Details of this evaluation have been presented elsewhere (43).

TABLE V

TARGETS

LATERAL THALAMOTOMY	(Voa - Vop - Zi)	36 cases
LATERAL and POSTERIOR THALAMOTOMY	(Pul-LP Complex)	12 cases

UNILATERAL THALAMOTOMIES 28	BILATERAL THALAMOTOMIES 8

The postoperative results were rated on a final score, which was the sum of the scores for the neurological and neurofunctional assessments. Each score was on a scale of 0 to 4. For the neurological assessment, 4-3-2 denoted respectively a very good-good-fair reduction of the symptom, 1 denotes a slight reduction and 0 mean no change or clinical deterioration. For the neurofunctional assessment, 0 denoted no improvement in performance in any of the four tests (global motor status, autonomy, grasp, tracing), 1 means improvement in at least one of the tests, 2 means improvement in two tests, 3 in three and 4 in all tests.

The final scores corresponded to the following degrees of improvement: 6-8 = very good (+++), 4-6 = good (++), 2-4 = fair (+), 1-2 = minimal (±) and 0 = no change (-). Table VI presents these improvements.

TABLE IV

IMPROVEMENT

IMPROVEMENT	N° OF PATIENTS
+++ (very good)	15
++ (good)	11
+ (fair)	10
± (minimal)	9
- (no change)	1

As shown in Figure 1, the best results were obtained in the cases with unilateral neurological signs in comparison with those with bilateral symptoms. In the former, in fact, both reduction of abnormal movements and increase of function were achieved. In the latter, however, some relief of the most disabling symptoms (such as dystonic movements or large excursion hyperkinesias), with a consequent improvement of existing functions, was not accompanied by additional functional capacities.

These considerations are strongly reflected in the tetraparetic cases with cerebral palsy, but also comply with cases with generalized Idiopathic Dystonia.

In these latter cases, in fact, the favourable results depend almost exclusively on the relief of the action tremor, combined with dystonic postures or action dystonia.

As shown in Figure 2, the most responsive symptoms were dystonic movements and large excursion hyperkinesias.

Action tremor always responded optimally to surgical treatment.

The dystonic postures, instead, had a variable reduction and in all cases this relief was less than that achieved in dystonic movements.

In regard to the distribution of the dystonias, those of the limb (absolutely prevalent in childhood) responded to surgical treatment, while those of the trunk (rare in childhood) were not modified.

186

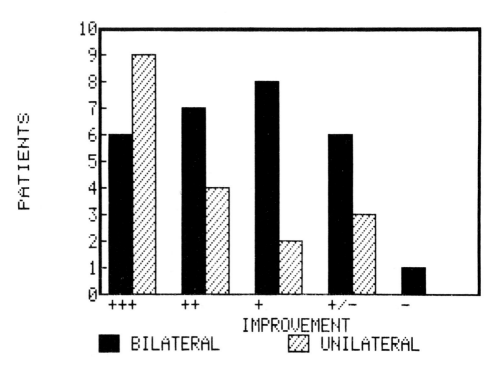

Fig. 1. Improvement versus distribution of symptoms

Although sometimes side effects occurred after unilateral operations, they were definitively more frequent after bilateral lesions. So in cases when clinical features could be corrected only by a bilateral thalamotomy, this risk must be carefully considered and may constitute a contra-indication to the surgical approach.

The side effects, discussed elsewhere (44), were: motor impairment (contralateral hemiparesis, gaze deficit, partial 3rd nerve paresis, increase of homolateral abnormal movements); sensory impairment (paresthesias); mood alteration (depression); disturbances of verbal function (dysarthria, reduction of voice volume). The disturbances of speech followed lesions on the dominant hemisphere and aphonia was an exclusive consequence of bilateral lesions. Depression, never reported by other Authors, occurred rather frequently in our cases and, interestingly, only after left thalamotomies. The interpretation of this curious symptom is discussed in a previous report (45).

Most of the side effects were transient and receded in 5 to 30 days. More resistant were dysarthria and residual pyramidal deficit, which took, sometimes, 6 months to disappear. In 2 patients a light permanent deficit of gait remained and in 2 other patients a severe aphonia never vanished. All of these patients underwent bilateral thalamotomy.

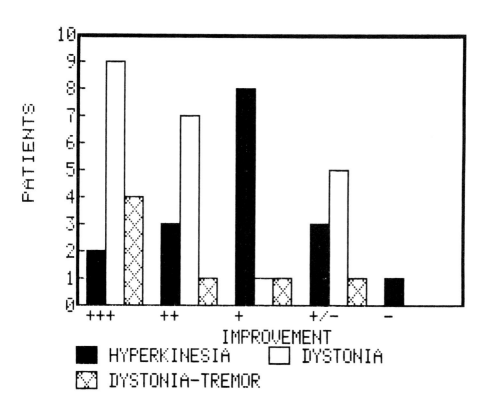

Fig. 2 Improvement versus different abnormal movements

188

CONCLUSIONS

Surgical therapy of abnormal movements in general and of dystonias in particular, must not be considered as the sole treatment, but as part of a combined therapy.

This combined treatment comprises drug therapy and surgical therapy, according to the progression of the symptoms and the degree of disability. The most recent information on the benefit of certain drugs (Levodopa, Trihexyphenidyl) in treatment of dystonias, render less indispensible or delay the surgical approach (46, 47, 48) for at least a certain number of cases. Surgical therapy is proposed in those cases in which the pharmacological treatment is not suitable (for example in action tremor), when this treatment stopped being effective or if the side effects supercede the benefits achieved.

The actual tendency, especially in the treatment of dystonias, is to initially attempt a pharmacological approach using a proposed sequence of drugs.

In our opinion, however, surgical approach can be the initial and exclusive therapeutic choice, in the treatment of certain clinical situations as in hemidystonias, combined or not combined with action tremor, because of the efficacy and scarcity of side effects.

This approach is considered advisable taking into consideration the young age of the patients and a consequence of chronic pharmacological treatment producing disturbing and often irreversible side effects.

ACKNOWLEDGEMENTS

This study was partially supported by the "Associazione Paolo Zorzi" for the Neuroscieces.

REFERENCES

1. Horsley V (1909) Brit Med J 124: 5-28
2. Meyers R (1940) Arch Neurol Psychiatr 44: 455-457
3. Bosch DA (1986) In: Stereotactic techniques in clinical neurosurgery. Springer Verlag, Wien-New York
4. Spiegel EA (1982) In: Guided brain operations. Karger, Basel
5. Spiegel EA, Wycis HT, Marks M, Lee AJ (1946) Science 106: 349-359
6. Spiegel AE, Wycis HT (1950) Arch Neurol Psychiatr 64: 295-296
7. Spiegel AE, Wycis HT (1954) Arch Neurol Psychiatr 71: 598-614
8. Cooper IS (1954) Science 119: 417-418
9. Hassler R (1955) In: Proceedings of the Second International Congress of

Neuropathology, Part 1. Excerpta Medica Foundation, Amsterdam, pp 29-40

10. Cooper IS, Bravo G, Riklan M, Duvoisin N, Gorek E (1958) Geriatrics 13: 127-147

11. Cooper IS (1969) Involuntary Movement Disorders. Hoeber Medical Division, New York

12. Cooper IS (1976) Advances in Neurology 14: 423-452

13. Mundinger F, Riechert T, Disselhoff J (1970) Conf. Neurol 32:71-78

14. Riechert T (1962) Conf Neurol 22: 356-363

15. Andrew J, Fowler CJ, Harrison MJG (1983) Brain 106: 981-1000

16. Anderson RL (1985) Advances in Ophthalmic Plastic and Reconstructive Surgery 4: 313-332

17. Battista AF (1985) Advances in Ophthalmic Plastic and Reconstructive Surgery 4: 369-377

18. Callahan A (1985) Advances in Ophthalmic Plastic and Reconstructive Surgery 4: 379-384

19. Fett DR, Putterman AM, Weingarten CZ (1985) Advances in Ophthalmic Plastic and Reconstructive Surgery 4: 349-360

20. Perman KI, Baylis HI (1985) Advances in Ophthalmic Plastic and Reconstructive Surgery 4: 397-405

21. Shore JW (1985) Advances in Ophthalmic Plastic and Reconstructive Surgery 4: 333-347

22. Small RG (1985) Advances in Ophthalmic Plastic and Reconstructive Surgery 4: 385-395

23. Wilkins RB, Bird WA (1985) Advances in Ophthalmic Plastic and Reconstructive Surgery 4: 361-368

24. Tsui JK, Eisen A, Mak E, Carruthers J, Scott AB, Calne DB (1985) Can J Neurol Sci 12: 314-316

25. Brin MF, Fahn S, Moskowitz C, Friedman A, Shale HM, Greene PE et al. (1987) Adv Neurol in press

26. Waltz JM (1982) In: Marsden CD, Fahn S (eds) Movement Disorders. Butterworths, London, pp 300-307

27. Goetz CG, Penn RD, Tanner CM (1987) Advances in Nerology in press

28. Kelly JP (1985) In: Kandel ER, Schwartz JH (eds) Principles of Neural Science. Elsevier, New York

29. Hassler R (1959) In: Einfuhrung in die stereotaktisschen Operationen mit einem Atlas des menschlinchen Gehirns. Vol I. Thieme, Stuttgart, pp. 230-290

30. Cooper IS (1957) JAMA 164:1297-1301

31. Narabayashi H (1962) Conf. Neurol 22: 364-367

32. Laitinen LV (1970) J Neurol Neurosurg Psychiatry 33:513-518

33. Siegfried J (19970) Rev Otoneuroophtalmol 42: 412-414

34. Balasubramanian V, Kanada TS, Ramanujam PB (1974) J Neurosurg 40: 577-582

35. Gornall P, Hitchcock E, Kirkland IS (1975) Dev Med Chil Neurol 17: 279-286

36. Cooper IS, Riklan M, Amin I, Waltz JM, Cullinan MA, Neurology 26: 744-753

37. Gros C, Frerebeau P, Perez-Dominguez E, Bazin M, Privat JM (1976) Neurochirurgia (Stuttgart) 19: 171-178

38. Broggi G, Angelini L, Bono R, Nardocci N, Oleari G (1981) Med Hyg 39: 2022-2030

39. Broggi G, Angelini L, Bono R, Giorgi C, Nardocci N, Franzini A (1983) Neurosurgery 12: 195-202

40. Avanzini G, Spreafico R, Broggi G, Giovannini P, Franceschetti S (1977)

Neurosci Lett 4: 135–143

41. Spreafico R, Kirk C, Franceschetti S, Avanzini G (1980) Exp Brain Res 40: 209 220

42. Broggi G, Fedrizzi E (1978) Med Hyg 36: 2046–2050

43. Broggi G, Angelini L, Nardocci N (1985) In: Siegfried J, Lazorthes Y, Broggi G (eds) La neurochirurgie fonctionnelle de l'infirmité motrice d'origine cérébrale Neurochirurgie 31 Suppl

44. Broggi G, Angelini L, Giorgi C (1980) Neurosurgery 7: 127–134

45. Angelini L, Nardocci N, Bono R, Broggi G (1982) Ital J Neurol Sci 3: 301–310

46. Marsden CD, Marion MH, Quinn N (1984) J Neurol Neurosurg Psychiatry 47: 1166–1173

47. Fahn S (1983) Neurology 33: 1255–1261

48. Fahn S, Marsden CD (1987) In: Marsden CD, Fahn S (eds) Movement Disorders 2 Butterworths, London, pp 359–382

Author Index